Nursing Replay

Nursing Replay
Researching Nursing Culture Together

Annette Street BEd(Hons) PhD
Post-Graduate Co-ordinator
Department of Nursing
La Trobe University
Melbourne, Australia

Honorary Research Fellow
Royal Children's Hospital Research Foundation
Melbourne, Australia

Honorary Research Associate
Department of Nursing
Victoria University at Wellington
Wellington, New Zealand

CHURCHILL LIVINGSTONE
MELBOURNE EDINBURGH LONDON MADRID NEW YORK TOKYO 1995

CHURCHILL LIVINGSTONE
An imprint of Pearson Professional

Pearson Professional (Australia) Pty Ltd
Kings Gardens
95 Coventry Street
South Melbourne 3205 Australia

First edition 1995

National Library of Australia Cataloguing-in-Publication Data

Street, Annette, 1948- .
    Nursing replay : researching nursing culture together.

    Bibliography.
    Includes index.
    ISBN 0 443 04761 8.

    1. Nursing – Research. 2. Nursing – Philosophy.
    I. Title.

    610.73072

Produced by Churchill Livingstone in Melbourne
through Longman Malaysia, VVP

For Churchill Livingstone in Melbourne
Publisher: Judy Waters
Editorial: Pam Jonas
Copy Editing: John Macdonald
Desktop Preparation: Sandra Tolra
Typesetting: Friedo Ligthart/Designpoint
Indexing: Max McMaster
Production Control: Robert Stagg
Design: Churchill Livingstone

The
publisher's
policy is to use
**paper manufactured
from sustainable forests**

Contents

Preface

This book replays unpublished work of the last four years on nursing culture discovered through my part in participatory clinical nursing research. New material has also been included which revisits the issues and ideas I have debated and discussed with nursing colleagues and students from Australia and overseas.

This book is not a recipe book but rather one exploring the lessons learnt establishing interactive participatory research designs in nursing practice. *Nursing Replay* examines the value of participatory research processes to enable us to better understand and bring about changes in nursing.

Participatory research is always contextualised research. Much of the research described in this book was carried out during the three years I was Director of the Centre for Studies in Paediatric Nursing (CSPN) at the Royal Children's Hospital (RCH) in Melbourne, Australia. The creation of the CSPN occurred as a result of my appointment to the RCH as a consultant to develop nursing research. There was no recognised model for a program with the objective of developing participatory research activities with clinical nursing staff. Without a blueprint, research staff had to learn by trial and error rather than by imitation and mentorship. As in most hospitals, the Royal Children's Hospital research community is heavily oriented to medical research. The needs and structures of medical research are often not compatible with qualitative or participatory research methods which can be useful for nursing. This difference in focus and methods means that nursing research is often without the infrastructure and external support available to the medical research community.

The work of the CSPN staff uncovered a number of concerns which proved to be consistent with the issues of establishing a research culture and community in any large institution. This book illustrates many of the research achievements along with some of the dilemmas and constraints.

The clinical nursing research staff were mainly novice researchers who had to learn about the processes while taking the responsibility for inducting others into research.

We all made mistakes. In order to raise the awareness of staff to the possibilities of nursing research while attempting to meet administrative needs, too many projects were initiated. Although these fledgling projects provided some knowledge and skills for the participants many did not reach publication. Some nurses in the clinical units had unattainable goals for nursing research. Others found it difficult to sustain enthusiasm when the processes took longer than they had expected and their colleagues did not appear to appreciate the fruits of their labors. The development of ward based research activities proved difficult in a culture governed by time constraints, shift work, and myths and misconceptions about the value of nursing research. Reluctantly the CSPN was closed in July 1993 due to budget cuts and a decision by senior management to develop clinical nursing research activities in a form which was integrated with a clinical school affiliated with a university school of nursing and the RCH Research Foundation. However the success of the work of the Centre was recently demonstrated when a meeting of sixty clinical nurses met with the executive staff to argue for the continuation of their research opportunities. As many other nurses were unable to attend because they were providing care for seriously ill children, this number represented a substantive commitment to clinical nursing research by the clinical nurses themselves. This show of interest and determination by nurses has been rewarded with support from administrative and medical staff and the allocation of funds for a nursing research program. The hospital board has also supported the proposition from the RCH nurses for higher degree programs in child health. The hospital has affiliated with the University of Melbourne to establish a clinical graduate program based at the hospital headed by a professor of child health nursing. The number and quality of presentations to the 1994 international conference in paediatric nursing derived from the research of the RCH nurses demonstrated the long term value of this developmental approach.

The experiences of my colleagues and I in the CSPN have propelled us on to the biggest learning curve of our lives. This book is the fruit of my own learning curve.

However the book would not have been written if I had not had the fortune to have been conducting research with many clinical nurses whose voices fill the pages of this book. The speaking voices of the nurses have been edited—a decision taken on the advice of my publisher because this is a book to be read and not a research project where every 'um' and 'ah' and the inconsistencies of everyday speech carry meaning. The editing has been done to carry the sense of conversations to the written page although I trust that the individual flavour of the quotes has been retained. In this sense it is a modernist production—a book which carries the stamp of the author as the decisions to include, omit and interpret the different voices of nurses and scholars are mine. Although I recognise that the post modern debates on the 'death of the author' mean that the text becomes open to a multiplicity of readings by the reader (Foucault 1977).

The early chapters are not research reports. Rather I have used the research data from a number of projects on specific topics and given it a theoretical reading. I have treated all the individual projects as part of a larger ethnographic study on the development of participatory research processes and explored them to illuminate and critique aspects of nursing culture.

Nursing Replay is also a tribute to the power of research partnerships with very special people. I am deeply indebted to those nurses whose work has informed mine and who have allowed me to use their anonymous stories here. I also acknowledge the contribution to the clarification of my thinking which my graduate students have provided over the last few years with their energetic questioning, their generous sharing of interesting papers and ideas, and their commitment to the discipline of nursing.

The work of Andrew Robinson and Jeanine Blackford at the Royal Children's Hospital was invaluable to the nursing staff with whom they worked and to me. The hours of debate and discussion, tears and laughter have taught us all many lessons about ourselves, about the research act and about the cultural practices of nursing. I continue to be very close friends with both Andrew and Jeanine and have the challenge and privilege to be supervising their doctoral work.

Likewise trans-Tasman research projects with Chris Walsh over the last twelve months have been a creative and educative experience. Chris is a talented researcher who has been a guide through the various aspects of cultural life in New Zealand, introducing me to important contacts in her wide web of con-nections. She has intelligence, wit, organisational skills, useful knowledge, a wonderful dog and great friends—and I have benefited from all these.

So with genuine gratitude I dedicate this book to three researchers who have been with me through the tough times and whom I love dearly—Jeanine, Andrew and Chris.

Introduction

Nursing is task-centred. I don't care what anyone says—it's tasks, tasks, tasks. We are here to look after the patients and to follow the doctors' orders. I can't see any value in sitting around talking about what we want to do, we just need to get on with it!

Jenny, an experienced nurse was initially very skeptical about participatory action research and the idea that nurses could improve patient care by investigating and restructuring their practice. The process known as participatory action research (PAR) is a valuable form of research for situations where the research topic is focused on issues of concern to practitioners and systematic and informed action is required. It is change oriented research which is interventionist and therefore political.

After hearing more about PAR Jenny was persuaded to join a research group. Later she wrote this account of an experience which demonstrated her changed attitude to the doctors and to the PAR process.

Daniel was 12 hours old when he was admitted. He was placed under an Ohio overhead heater which enables newborn babies to be nursed exposed with overhead temperature regulation. Daniel was stripped of all clothing. When I walked in I saw the baby was crying lustily, all limbs were thrashing, and he was bright red and very distressed. There were two doctors and one nurse present concentrating on deciding a diagnosis and getting ready to insert an intravenous line as he needed instant prostaglandin. I looked at him and thought 'Oh that poor baby, just born straight from the security of the womb, now under bright lights and no mother to hold him'. I decided to see what would happen if I cuddled the baby under one hand and stroked his brow with the other and spoke to him in low soothing tones. The doctors proceeded talking and taking little interest (well perhaps only technical interest) in the baby and the nurse was setting up the intravenous tray and fluid. The baby calmed very quickly as I spoke to him, heart and respiratory rate dropped dramatically and he lay still. The doctor, was able to insert the IV into the baby's arm without any undue restraint of the arm and without any anxiety on the part of the baby. The doctor said to me 'What are you doing, I need strapping!'

I said: 'I'm looking after the baby's emotional needs!' He was a tall man leaning under the Ohio overhead heater and he said: 'Well, we need strapping and my head's getting burnt!' So I sang out for someone else to get him strapping. Daniel did not even move, he stayed absolutely still, heart and respiratory rates stayed stable and he appeared comfortable. I sang out for someone to get him a dummy because I thought 'Well I couldn't stand here all afternoon stroking his head'. We got a dummy in and tucked a nappy around him to settle him down and he was fine.

These are the interesting things for me. Afterwards one nurse said: 'Oh, you're showing off, just trying to get out of work'. Another nurse was so fascinated that she recorded this incident in her own journal, but the doctor was irritated that I wouldn't cut the strapping for him and help run the IV through. He saw the technical task as a priority and he thought that I was there to assist him not to care for the baby's emotional needs.

The reason I decided to concentrate purely on the emotional angle was because of the work of the action research group which I am involved with where we are looking at paediatrics from a nursing perspective. The experience of being in this action research group has changed my practice and made me really look carefully at things. I am fascinated at the difference it makes when you stop and think. You need to be fairly comfortable though and not get caught up in the technical tasks.

Jenny's experience with PAR has changed her understanding of nursing and the possibilities for the care she provides. Others around her have noticed and commented on the difference in her approach.

Nursing Replay represents the potential of participatory forms of research to replay the drama of nursing practice through reflection and deconstruction and then replay collaboratively the action through processes of reconstruction.

All forms of participatory research must be developed reciprocally between the researchers and the participants. Generally the participants are the researchers and can be labelled 'researchers', 'research participants' or 'co-researchers'. In participatory research the findings need to be disseminated in such a form that the participants, and others in their situation, can understand and use them (Lather 1991). In this way the findings are directed at the people involved in the situation rather than at the academic or research community. This was apparent in a participatory project in which I was invited to join with members of the Denver project in Colorado. The project director Ruth Neil and some of the HIV positive men had joined together to discover how to represent what hope meant for them for a poster display to be presented at the International Caring Conference. The group made decisions about the images which could be used to represent their experiences using a participatory research process. The findings in the form of a poster display of their own special photos was presented to the other HIV positive people in the project and to the international nursing community.

These kinds of participatory research emphasise collaborative exploration and are fed by feminist critiques of the isolated and elitist position taken by the objective researcher in relation to those who are being researched. Harding (1986) argues that feminist inquiry of the natural and social world is an intervention of political and moral illumination.

The process of engaging in practices which are informed by *PRAXIS* reflection is called *praxis*. Praxis is a political process where reasoning and action mutually inform each other. Praxis research is based on the premise that research is not neutral. As Lather comments: 'Research approaches inherently reflect our beliefs about the world we live in and want to live in' (Lather 1991:51).

Praxis research strategies value reciprocity in research relationships, negotiation of meaning and theorising which speaks to the understandings and conditions of the participants (Lather 1991). These strategies are directed at identifying the complexity of practice through the identification of issues which arise from an area of concern to the participants. The research focus on issues rather than on problems enables the participants to examine the situation from a number of angles. Problem focused research assumes that the problem is known and so the researchers focus in a pre-determined way. Issues can be explored as they emerge within the process and can be addressed concurrently through policy, social organisation and practice.

Participatory forms of research are now taking their place alongside other equally useful research. Nurses need to be involved in other people's research and to read and use other people's research findings. But also the challenge is for nurses to participate in their own research. In the document 'Adversity and Child Health A Strategy for Policy-Directed Research' the major findings include the statement regarding

> the importance of non-hierarchical participative research methodologies is recognised, particularly as far as research into the experiences of children and parents or the planning of community projects is concerned. It is argued, however, that there are other valuable research areas in which traditional empirical methods may be more appropriate. The important point is that methodologies are consistent with the project in hand, and that projects are consistent with the principle of equity (p. viii).

This statement, with its affirmation of the value of non-hierarchical participatory research and its plea that the research community do not disregard traditional empirical methods, is very interesting. It places participatory or praxis research in a normative position in relation to other research.

Praxis research owes a significant theoretical debt to critical theory (Habermas 1971, Fay 1977, 1987). It is informed by a critical concern to identify issues and collaborate to reflect politically upon practice to systematically reconstruct it. Critical theory presumes that individuals can make rational choices and act to improve a given situation. This assumption is part of the modern world view that there are some basic foundational ethics and that individuals can critique their experiences against universal criteria of rationality and justice.

The understanding and action component of critical theory fits well with nursing practice. Nurses become nurses because they want to be involved in healing—an active process—and one which enables them not only to understand a given situation, but also to do something about it. Participatory research arises from a belief that groups of people can find general agreement about what is just and necessary in certain situations and about how to act ethically in that context. This view assumes that it is possible to decode situations and to decide what is 'just'. Critics of this modernist idea challenge the underlying assumption that there is a universally accepted notion of 'justice' or 'right' or 'ethical action' which is independent from the culturally constructed beliefs of a group of people. One of the key arguments of this post modern critique is from post structural theorists who have demonstrated that language not only expresses what we can think or say, but limits and shapes what it is possible for us to think or say. This critique challenges the idea that a group of people can understand and reconstruct their situation from a position which is 'emancipatory' to others.

The participatory work of Paulo Freire (1972) has been developed further through critical pedagogy (McLaren 1988, Luke & Gore 1992, Lather 1991). Although critical pedagogy emerges from the modern position, the major proponents of this approach share the post modern interest in deconstructing the power relations inherent in our discursive positions. I share this post modern interest in language and discourse (e.g. Spivak 1990, Weedon 1987) which along with the concepts of space imparted by post modern geography (e.g. Rose 1993) architecture (e.g. Colomina 1992, Spain 1992) and the interests of cultural studies (e.g. Minh-ha 1991, Moraga & Anzaldua 1983) currently informs my changing understandings. I also share with Thompson (1991) an interest in participatory feminist nursing research on race, gender and sexuality.

In this book the emphasis will be on exploring PAR, journalling and other forms of praxis research through a lens in which the critical, feminist and post modern forms of research are in tension with each other. This is not an eclectic position as I do not take bits of different theories to remake them as a coherent theory. Rather, it is an attempt to make a space in the margins which allows me to use the strategies and theoretical underpinning of both these modernist and post modernist positions to unsettle the ideas and actions I develop while in either.

Critical feminist thought is directed at using a process of reflection to understand the power relationships and imbalances in the experiences of the participants and then at acting to redress them. This process of knowledge generation is described by Haraway (1988) as 'power sensitive conversations'. Fine (1992:227) describes 'participatory activist' research as 'at once disruptive, transformative, and reflective; about understanding and about action; not about freezing the scene but always about change'.

Post structuralist feminist processes of deconstruction remind us that the world is a place of multiple and contradictory views and decision making processes (Weedon 1987). Weedon (1987:8) argues for the role of the 'subjective' because 'the ways people make sense of their lives is a necessary starting point for understanding how power relations structure society'. People experience themselves as 'subjects' who are unable to be simply categorised as a 'nurse' or 'woman' or 'partner' or 'researcher' or 'neighbor' or 'friend', but know themselves as all these things at the same time.

Subjectivity is constituted historically as a product of our society and culture and at any given time some of these 'subject positions' will be dominant. At work a person may be a researcher who at any moment can act out of any of these multiple subject positions which are informed by any number of discourses. Post structural feminists remind us that none of us represent the essential 'woman' or 'nurse' or 'administrator'. In any given situation we will act to exercise power or have power exercised upon us in response to the complexities of the situation and within the range of possibilities open to us as individuals (Spivak 1990). Nurses find themselves continually enmeshed in contradictory and fluid power relations with medical staff, patients and clients, their families and significant others, and with other members of staff. Research with nurses needs to take account of these relationships as well as highlight the power relations exercised in the context by the presence and interventions of the researchers themselves.

Post structural thinking challenges any notions we may have about using participatory research processes to find a single true and right answer or the correct course of action. Forms of post structural research acknowledge that conclusions are multiple, contradictory and partial rather than definitive. The emergent, tentative understandings need to be checked out time and again with the participants in a reciprocal process. There is a need to accept that a decision made in one context may not be right for all time or even for other places, but is a decision that fits the needs of those participants at that particular time, place and context.

Critical research processes, when 'interrogated' by post structural analyses, carry the potential to enable people who want to improve their situation to not only deconstruct it but to attempt to change things (Lather 1992). As Lykes (1989:179) suggests

it affirms a commitment on the part of both researcher and participant to engage the research process as subjects, as constructors of our own reality.

Participatory research attempts to break the silences which have controlled the way research is done and to challenge the view of what is 'natural' or 'scientific' (Harding 1986, Haraway 1988). Participatory researchers seek to discover ways of knowing and acting which are not mainstream and framed by the dominant discourses of life; and to track down and emphasise those experiences which exist in the margins (Stanley & Wise 1993, de Lauretis 1988, Weedon 1987).

In writing as a feminist who as yet cannot manage to research exclusively within either the empowering praxis of modernity or the deconstructive strategies of post structuralism, I see myself as researching on the margins. I work with participatory research while challenging the limitations of its modernist history. I think that praxis research has something important to offer nurses investigating nursing.

Research is constructed as a modernist exercise. The concept of a logical argument and a structure imposed by modernist research conventions which culminate in findings of some sort is antithetical to post modern positions. I have difficulty as yet conceptualising how to use post structuralist and post modern strategies developed for texts, images and buildings, to develop the texts-in-action of dynamic political research with people. As Spivak said in an interview with Harasym (1988), the strategies of deconstruction cannot *ground* politics. In research with people I can deconstruct after the interventionist research strategy but I can't engage in participatory research and label what I do post modern. However the conceptual ideas and the products of work from the natural sciences and post modern arts provide a rich intellectual resource of knowledge and strategies which 'trouble' the reflexive and participatory research processes I engage in with nurses.

THE CALL FOR CLINICAL NURSING RESEARCH

The nursing literature since Florence Nightingale is replete with pleas for nurses to engage in research on nursing issues and practices (for example, see Allen 1985, Allen & Benner et al 1986, Chaska 1978, Fawcett 1984, Gortner 1983, Greenwood 1984, Chinn 1986, Hunt 1987). The fact that the pleas continue indicates that few nurses engage in clinical research because it is not considered a mainstream activity as it is for their medical colleagues.

There are some models where nursing research is directly developed by clinical nurses and used in the clinical area. One is at The Children's Hospital at Denver. The Kempe Research Centre is located there and integrated with the nearby School of Nursing at the University of Colorado (Keefe 1993). The centre was established to foster high quality nursing research which is clinically relevant and beneficial to children (Keefe & Kotzer 1988). The aim of the centre is to integrate research findings into nursing practice through an integrated research utilisation model which is based on the work of four committees. The research committee identifies clinical problems to be researched, assembles and critiques and summarises the relevant literature. If the review suggests that a replication study would be useful then this can be carried out through the work and support of the research committee. The procedure committee revises procedures and policies in the light of research findings and develops new protocols. The education committee develops standardised care educational reference tools and offers in-service education while the quality assurance committee monitors the implementation of change strategies and measures patient outcomes. The centre's research program is built up around professional researchers doing research with a strong organisation to make sure that the nursing research is relevant to practice and utilised by clinicians. This nursing research implementation program is valuable in many ways. It does not intentionally assist clinical nurses to develop their own research skills or to participate actively in the research except as data collectors or implementors.

YOU MUST DO CLINICAL RESEARCH— IT'S IN YOUR JOB DESCRIPTION!

In Australia the emergence of job descriptions for nurses has provided the instrument to specify that nurses engage in research. In Queensland job descriptions for all levels contain a requirement for nurses to engage in action research. However Queensland Health has not provided the infrastructure or skilled support for nurses to learn how to do action research, neither has it provided the time for them to do it. Fortunately for the nurses who inherited these job descriptions, their performance appraisals do not hold them accountable for their research productivity as action researchers. Endeavors like these are pointless unless the infrastructure support, education and resources are provided to make rhetoric a reality.

The most promising initiative in Australia has been the development of professorial nursing research units. These units began in England and the concept and structure was introduced into Australia by Professor Alan Pearson when he established the School of Nursing at Deakin University, Geelong. Professorial nursing research units enable academic nurses to hold joint university and hospital appointments and establish research and nursing practices in the institutional unit. The units however usually need to work at acquiring and conducting fundable research, which often doesn't allow time or resources for the development of research skills in other clinical staff in the institution.

THE CENTRE FOR STUDIES IN PAEDIATRIC NURSING

The Centre for Studies in Paediatric Nursing aimed to assist nursing staff in meeting the needs of hospitalised children and their families. In order to do so the nursing research was constituted to meet three interconnected objectives:

1. To develop research which is directed to better understanding the needs of children and their families.
2. To engage nursing staff in research which enables them to examine and reconstruct their own nursing practice in order to better meet the needs of children and their families.
3. To teach nursing staff to develop the skills necessary to design and conduct their own research projects related to clinical practice and to be able to write their findings for the use of the wider nursing community through publication.

This research centre required a critical mass of infrastructure staff. Two hospital Clinical Nurse Specialist Teachers were seconded to the newly created Clinical Nurse Researcher positions. The hospital provided office and meeting space, secretarial support, computers and related facilities and a small budget for some equipment, furniture, books and stationery.

The staff of the CSPN focused on developing small unit-based research activities with clinical nurses and with facilitating the development of the skills, knowledge and the research experience of staff from those areas. During 1991-92 the CSPN engaged in three small externally funded projects which added four researchers to the team. The CSPN became a satellite centre of La Trobe University and two collaborative research projects were funded externally in conjunction with the La Trobe Centre for Research in Public Health and Nursing. Key research was in the areas of asthma, pain management, nursing children with disabilities, patient education, breastfeeding, the nursing management of children with cardiac anomalies and the interface between the hospital and the community (see Blackford 1993, Robinson et al 1993, Robinson & O'Connell 1994, Parsons et al 1994a &1994b). The staff of the CSPN also engaged in consultancies with other hospitals and university departments throughout Australia, spoke at conferences, conducted workshops, marked theses, and supervised student research.

The valuable research work of the CSPN staff and the nurse participants is evident throughout the book. During the life of the CSPN I continued to hold a part time appointment as a Senior

Lecturer at the Department of Nursing at La Trobe university. The clinical nursing researchers continued to work in the units where they had formerly been clinical teachers. After negotiation with the unit managers, these units were attached to the Centre. These units formed a major focus of the research activity although other units became involved. The latest PAR project at the RCH involved all units and was conducted in conjunction with other hospitals and the Victorian Health Promotion Foundation.

THE SHAPE OF THE BOOK

The first chapters of this book explore some aspects of nursing culture, both as a backdrop to the research, and as an illumination of the cultural practices which have emerged through the process of analysis and reflection during the research. These analyses have not been written as research accounts. They are part of my wider feminist deconstruction of the theoretical insights from individual participatory projects in which I have been involved over the last four years.

I write both as scholar and participant, researcher and re-searched, a colluder in nursing culture and yet critic of it, an author who takes on the authority to interrogate the voices, one who is silenced as a 'non-nurse', and a woman who inhabits privileged and marginal spaces at the same time. My own voice changes throughout the text. Sometimes I write as a group member whose insights are represented as 'we'; at other times I write my own critique as 'I'; and at other times I place myself outside the situation and write about 'the nurses'. These changes may not always be comfortable for the reader but represent an attempt to reflect the participatory nature of some of the insights and action. They also represent my attempt to 'own' my own insights and values. Porter (1993) argues that this is uncommon in nursing scholarship because of a mistaken quest for objectivity:

> Asserting the effects of the researcher upon the research is not merely a meta-theoretical quibble; it is of considerable practical significance, affecting profoundly the way in which reports are regarded (Porter 1993:140).

The voices of those people reported in this book also jostle for position and are privileged over the voices I chose to ignore, or could not hear because the power I exercised by my very presence silenced them. In keeping with my commitment to the valuing of both academic scholarship and nursing practice the voices of scholars do not drown the voices of nurses. Theoretical ideas and practical examples are juxtaposed to show their complementarity and contrasts.

Chapter 1 explores some of the myths of nursing and charts their relationship to clinical practice. This chapter is a reworking of a plenary paper entitled Nursing Myths in Action which was presented to the 4th National Nursing Education Conference, Myth, Mystery and Metaphor held in November, 1990 in Melbourne, Australia. This paper was written during the early stages of this four year period and has evolved with further experience on theorising and engaging in participatory research (Street 1990c).

The second chapter entitled Being Caring: Getting Beyond the Tyranny of Niceness is a reworking of another plenary paper of the same name presented to the 14th International Caring Conference, Human Caring: A Global Agenda on July 8th 1992, in Melbourne, Australia. Caring is an integral part of the scholarship and practice of nursing. It is an area which has often been written about but which has sustained little critique (see Walker 1993).

The concepts of time and space are explored in Chapter 3 through their relationship to clinical nursing practice. This work was foreshadowed in an earlier book (Street 1992a) but I have begun a more extensive analysis here because I consider that we have given precedence to notions of time over space and to linearity over mapping (Street 1993b).

The remaining chapters are devoted to investigations of participatory forms of clinical research. Participatory action research is discussed in some detail as it is the form of participatory research most commonly used in our work at the Royal Children's Hospital.

In writing about the PAR process I have not chosen to reproduce information on 'how to do action research' as there are entire books and chapters in books devoted to this form of explanation (see Webb 1989, 1991, Wadsworth 1991, Tripp 1990, Carr 1989, Carr & Kemmis 1986, McTaggart 1991a &1991b, Reason 1988, van Manen 1990, Whyte 1991).

This is not a book debating the merits of action research nor an in-depth analysis of its historical and theoretical roots, however I would like to present Wadsworth's (1991) explanation of PAR:

> Participatory action research is not just research which we hope will be followed by action! It is action which is researched, changed and re-researched within the research process. Nor is it simply an exotic variation of consultation. Instead it is active co-research, by and for those who are to be helped. Nor can it be used by one group of people to get another group of people to do what is thought best for them—

whether that is to implement a central policy or an organisational or service change. Instead it is a genuinely democratic process whereby those to be helped, determine the purposes and outcomes of their own inquiry. Paradoxically it is quite close to a commonsense way of going about 'learning by doing'. But at the same time it is very hard to achieve the ideal conditions for putting it fully into practice (Wadsworth 1991:1).

This description of PAR encapsulates a way of thinking about participatory research which is consistent with my own theoretical leanings. It re-positions the concerns in the hands of those involved—regardless of whether the concerns appear trivial or traumatic to an outside party. Although no one wants to expend a great deal of energy on the trivial sometimes it is easier for novice researchers to chose something relatively simple so they can focus on acquiring some research skills. Often the trivial rapidly leads to the complex as it is the tip of the iceberg.

Many of the books and articles on action research written from a nursing perspective have been concerned with action research as a management process for change. In these projects the researcher has been either a participant-observer (Shea 1979) an educator (Webb 1990, McCaugherty 1991) or a collaborator (Smith 1986). In this book I am attempting to illustrate how nurse researchers using the process have made their research decisions in the context of their ongoing clinical or academic practice. I have identified some of the strategies nurses have found helpful in order to develop the skills and knowledge necessary to conduct the research and to find a way through the dilemmas and pitfalls they have encountered along the way.

The PAR process shares common assumptions and practices with action research as it is used in other disciplines in education and the social sciences. However, in recognition of the distinctiveness of the discipline of nursing, this process has been structured and re-structured through collaboration with nursing colleagues. In designing the process I initially borrowed heavily from the original Deakin University Faculty of Education Action Research Planner written by Stephen Kemmis and Robin McTaggart (1982). However the shape of the process has evolved through constant implementation and modification.

In Chapter 5 I describe the process as I use it with nurses in order to inform other nurses and academics who may be interested in tailoring PAR to meet their own situation in the manner that Arphorn Chuaprapaisilip (1990) has adapted the action research process to incorporate the Buddhist teaching (Satpatthana) for nurses in Thailand.

Most conventional forms of social research are directed at the development of information concerning a question or hypotheses, posed by a researcher or group, for application in practice by another group of people. So they make clear distinctions between the categories of researchers or theorists from those who experience the problem in their personal or professional lives. In contrast, PAR conflates these distinctions between the researchers and the researched, involving both groups together in the research process. Those people who will be most directly affected by the research 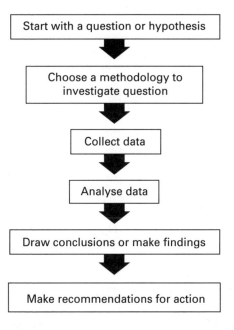and who may be required to live with its consequences are considered as the critical reference group. As such they are involved in the entire research process from problem formulation to final evaluation. Participatory action research is done with and for them— they become participatory researchers with all its attendant contradictions (Connors 1988).

Another distinction between conventional research designs and the design of a PAR project is in the structure of the research. Conventional research designs can be charted in a linear form where each stage has its distinctive position (see Fig. 1.1).

Start with a question or hypothesis

Choose a methodology to investigate question

Collect data

Analyse data

Draw conclusions or make findings

Make recommendations for action

Fig. 1.1 Conventional research design

The stages of conventional research designs follow each other inexorably. Once the hypotheses or question has been clearly established and the research design constructed and implemented there is no opportunity to go back and say:

Hey, we asked the wrong question—we want to change it in midstream.

Now that we know this we can't keep collecting data and leave the situation untouched—we want to act now and change the research design.

The question/situation has changed so we want to restructure the study.

As PAR is the method of choice when people want to understand and improve their situation, there is an expectation that the situation **will** change and that questions may need to be reformulated to meet the needs of the changed context. This creates the problem of how to illustrate the shape of the research design. Following Kurt Lewin (1946) the founder of action research, I use a design based on a corkscrew shape to demonstrate the open ended yet ongoing structure of a PAR project with an evaluation/reflection stage to facilitate problem reformulation or replanning of action. Although some nurses use a circular shape (e.g. East & Robinson 1994) I find that the corkscrew shape more effectively demonstrates the spaces and fluidity of the process as we use it (see Fig. 1.2).

I also want to emphasise that there is a difference between the kind of planned action which results from PAR and a meeting on ward issues or curriculum planning. To engage in research we need systematic data for analysis. We need to be able to stand back from the action with the kind of information that will give us a clear picture of what happened when the action was implemented. This evidence can be collected in a variety of ways using both qualitative and quantitative methods. The main aim is to make the data collection strategy match the action and where possible to use multiple data sources to provide a more complete picture.

I have conducted workshops on PAR throughout Australia, in the United States of America, in Hong Kong and in New Zealand. In each instance the same key issues were raised although the way that they effect practice is dependent on the particular context. While questions of resources in Australia may relate to outmoded cardiac monitors, in subtropical Hong Kong nurses reported that there were not enough blankets during a spell of very cold weather. A recent workshop in Australia, which involved nurses from clinical, administrative and academic settings, produced the following areas of concern:

THOSE MOST DIRECTLY AFFECTED BY THE Research
& WHO MAY BE REQUIRED TO LIVE
WITH IT'S CONSEQUENCES COMPRISE THE CRITICAL
Reference Group.'

useful

The participatory action research process

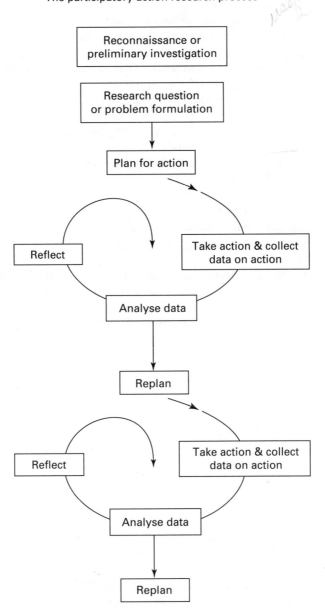

Fig. 1.2 The participatory action research process

- habitual practices and the difficulty of introducing lasting changes
- inequity in workloads
- patient rights and how to support them in the hospital setting
- the tension for academics between teaching and faculty practice
- the need for better community resources to refer patients to
- more effective patient assessments
- the lack of time for discharge education with reduced bed stay days
- the difficulty of providing privacy for patients in open wards
- the intrusion of ward rounds
- the dominance of medical knowledge over nursing knowledge and its effect on patient care
- doctor/nurse relationships
- nurse/nurse relationships
- ineffective communication between staff
- duplication of activities such as assessment by many health professionals
- the changed expectations of the nurse administrator's role
- the need for more effective pain management practices
- the problem of priority setting when the ward is task-focused
- the introduction of new nursing procedures
- the development of nursing protocols for new medical procedures
- role conflicts with extra responsibilities being added to job descriptions
- the need to keep current in nursing
- lack of resources for clinical nursing research
- the need for nursing input into decisions on the acquisition of new technology.

This list covers a wide range of nursing concerns and to become PAR topics they would need to be focused on a specific manageable aspect of the larger area of concern.

Although PAR is the major focus of this book it is only one of a number of reflective participatory research processes described. Chapter 7 provides an account of a related form of praxis research which is being conducted in New Zealand in conjunction with a New Zealand nurse researcher, Chris Walsh (Street & Walsh 1994b). This kind of participatory research is useful for researchers who are not working continually in the field as it is easier to manage in short sustained bursts and it is useful for those who want to develop a multi-site project. It is possible for this form of research to be set up to gain widespread validation from others who share the common concerns and to inform laws, policies, structures, education and make a contribution to practice.

Chapter 8 is a re-worked version of a small monograph I wrote on journalling which has found its way to various parts of the globe (Street 1990a). Following the work of Professor John Smyth (1986) I have always used journalling as not just a repository of stories, but as a research strategy for nurses.

Chapter 9 enables me to explore the experiences of being a participatory researcher using the voices of some of the nurses who have participated in research with me and the voices of my colleagues who have been employed as full time clinical researchers with a manifesto to develop participatory clinical research. Some of these ideas were originally presented as 'Launching into the Deep: Dealing with Doubts, Dilemmas and Despair', a conference address to Embodiment Empowerment Emancipation: Critical theory, reflectivity and nursing practice, held in Melbourne, on February 15-16 (Street, 1990b) and in a consultancy report (Street & Walsh, 1994a).

1. Noticing the unnoticed in clinical nursing practice

That's blue.
It's purple!
No I call that blue, that one's purple!
They are both purple and that's pink!
It's what I call purple!

These remarks were made by a group of graduate nursing students when I asked them to name a range of color shades from pink through to blue. The difficulty we had agreeing on a name for those blue hues with a pink/red tinge or pink hues with a blue tinge demonstrated how each person cut the color spectrum at different points. The decision appeared to depend upon what reinforcement each had received for their individual responses in the past. So the question of when blue or pink/red becomes purple was not a question about a universal given. It was an example of a temporarily allocated meaning which was person specific and context specific. This temporality became evident to the group members when the colors were juxtaposed against other similar shades.

Unless we are color blind we all see the color spectrum as a spectrum of graded hues without discrete boundaries. It is through the language and practices of our culture that we allocate boundaries to the color spectrum (Gee 1993). According to Gee some cultures use only four basic color terms, others use seven and English speaking cultures have eleven basic color terms. Each see the same colors but describes them differently.

We live lives constituted by meanings and taken for granted assumptions which shape the way we think and act. Nursing has its own discrete culture consisting of meanings, roles and rituals, myths and maxims, practices and theories which are distinctive and differentiate nursing from other health care cultures. Noticing the unnoticed in clinical nursing practice means making visible those aspects of nursing culture which have become taken for

1

granted and therefore 'invisible' to nurses. It means cutting the cultural spectrum of nursing in different ways to show habitual patterns of thinking and practising nursing.

Praxis research enables nurses to investigate the spectrum of their practice. The cultural spectrum can be cut in a number of different ways. In other books (see Street 1990d, 1991, 1992b, 1992c) I have cut the spectrum to examine clinical nursing histories, oral traditions, forms of embodiment, caring and gender. Although these aspects of nursing culture receive some treatment in this book I have specifically chosen to cut the nursing culture spectrum to disclose nursing myths in action, power relationships, and the aspects of time and space structuring clinical nursing. An exploration of these topics has emerged through a variety of participatory research projects which I have taken part in over the last four years. These projects were deliberately structured so that we not only investigated, acted and reflected upon the focus of the project but also on the wider implications for nursing through deconstruction of the interrelationships between practices, structures and policies.

THE POWER OF NURSING MYTHS IN ACTION

The power of myths in our lives cannot be underestimated. Healing occurs on many levels and for many reasons, yet concrete images of science and technology so dominate our western ways of thinking about healing that we often attribute to science a capacity for healing far beyond what it can possibly deliver. We become caught up in the myth of scientism, where the products and methods of science are accorded unacknowledged forms of authority over our thinking (Habermas 1971). Or we challenge all forms of science, and its products, and live with the myth that science is inherently dangerous—an attitude seen in some more extreme areas of natural therapies.

Symbolic meanings which are encapsulated in myths enter our psyche at a profoundly deep level—speaking to us in ways we do not often openly comprehend, and making claims on our actions in ways which we do not often acknowledge. The challenge is to locate, and regularly revisit, these submerged myths because they are generative of who we are and how we live our lives.

Myths are culturally created, containing elements acceptable to the members of a particular culture or cultural sub-group. The genesis of a myth within a cultural context is the basis for its power over members of that particular socio-cultural context, whereas members of an alternate cultural reality may find the same myth puzzling and eminently resistible.

COMPETING MYTHS CONSTRUCTED THROUGH CULTURE

Equally, scientific practices which shape our thinking are mythical to people from other cultures. In our western culture myths are generally disregarded as such; we relegate myths to other cultures and classify our world through 'facts'. However the elements of healing myths from other times and places are found in the healing myths of our own culture. There are a number of myths relating to health and illness, which may affect and shape nursing myths, but which transcend nursing culture and represent the concerns of all the members of the wider community who share a common cultural base. According to Moyers (1988:5):

> we all need to understand death and to cope with death, and we all need help in our passages from birth to life and then to death.

Nurses know that their work puts them in touch with some of these transitions which are represented in myths from all cultures. However a cultural blindness to the power of western science means that nurses may have little understanding of the power exercised by the myths of other cultures leading to incomprehension from both sides (Rice 1993). In a breastfeeding study, the nurses were amazed that colostrum, to them a highly prized creamy fluid available to the newborn baby prior to the onset of breast milk, was regarded as dirty pus by Vietnamese mothers. The nurses were horrified that the Vietnamese babies were being given pulped rice until the breast milk came in. In turn the Vietnamese mothers were horrified that the nurses wanted them to feed their baby with what they considered was a dirty, infected substance.

Nursing myths are also bound up in nursing culture and carry specific messages for nurses in ways that may be meaningless to other health care professionals. These nursing myths are generative of the practice of nurses and may specifically contain or imply a number of understandings or maxims. We can pursue this point by identifying and examining nursing myths which are full of such tacit understandings and implicit maxims.

THE TRADITIONAL NURSE OF MYTH

Nursing literature abounds with clear analyses of what I would like to label the traditional myth. I am using the word traditional here to refer to the historically created, taken for granted ideas of what and who a nurse is which have shaped nursing culture and which have been the subject of critical scrutiny by nurse scholars for years (e.g. Styles 1982, Pearson 1985, Henderson 1977, Chaska 1978, 1983).

This mythical nurse is born both female and nurse. She grows up as mother's little helper and daddy's little princess. Dressed in her miniature nurse uniform complete with obligatory veil/cap with red cross and matching red cape she tenderly tends her dolls, pets and friends through imaginary illnesses. She is very interested in cleanliness and tidiness and in selflessly caring for the needs and desires of other household members, particularly the males. Everyone knows she is a born nurse so she is encouraged to be kind rather than clever. She is middle-class, white and heterosexual. At the first chance her destiny is confirmed when she leaves school and is whisked off to the security of the nurse's home of her chosen hospital or to the classroom of her chosen university. Once ensconced there she is inaugurated into the mysteries of sponges, bed making and cleaning, activities which she must unlearn and re-learn in the prescribed manner. She is also initiated into the mysteries of science, carefully organised into lectures which reflect the medical curriculum, so that she learns about the body as a number of systems which can become dysfunctional and then cured by the use of drugs and technology overseen by the omniscient doctor. Under careful supervision she is trained into all the requisite attitudes, rituals and routines which shape and dominate the domain of the sick.

What does this mythical nurse do when she is trained? She looks after the doctors and the patients in specific pre-determined ways, that is, ways which have been pre-determined by her superiors. She learns that nurses are expected to collect data for doctors and nursing administration but 'real' nurses are too busy to write about their nursing practice either for themselves or to share with their colleagues (Street 1990b). In fact they are always busy doing routine tasks, or enforcing procedural rules which have been broken by other nurses lower on the hierarchy, or by patients and by their families. Doctors alone appear to remain above regulation by nurses. Our mythical nurse learns that 'real' nurses are always clinicians, who are essentially practical people. These clinical nurses are the ones who do all the real work while educators and administrators sit around talking, writing or going to meetings. These nurses also know that their role involves being seen always working hard finishing tasks, not sitting down talking to patients, a role filled by other health professionals, the charge nurse, or even the doctor. However our mythical nurse must endeavour to look neat and yet glamorous in an often ill fitting uniform in order to effectively play the 'doctor-nurse game' (Stein 1967).

Our mythical nurse happily inhabits a context of medical and administrative dominance; of oppression by gender, class, race and sexuality; of task-formed routines and rituals; of constant adaptability; and of childlike dependence on others to develop her further instruction; to take responsibility for her work; and to maintain her image as an angel of mercy. Her future is either virginally devoted to caring for the doctors, the hospital ward and the sick, or else involves marriage with a doctor enabling her to leave the hospital to care for the doctor, his household and his sick patients.

This, then, is the traditional myth of nurses and nursing which has been clearly exposed and repudiated in nursing literature. Nursing scholars have elucidated their own version of the mythical nurse, which I will call the myth of the professional nurse, but which could perhaps be subtitled the nurse educator's dream.

THE MYTHICAL PROFESSIONAL NURSE— THE NURSE EDUCATOR'S DREAM

This person is either male or female and enters a tertiary college or university program with strong marks in science and the arts. The student has deliberately chosen to enter a nursing course after careful consideration of all available career options. The professional nurse responds well to adult learning principles, cultivating a disciplined inquiring attitude to study and a healthy scepticism of irrational and hierarchically imposed cultural practices in nursing.

After graduation, professional nurses demonstrate a strong commitment to, and respect for their nursing colleagues and an ability to engage in assertive advocacy to ensure the best interest of the patient. They work co-operatively with medical and paramedical staff, sure of their own unique contribution to the health care team. They engage in effective documentation of their nursing actions and intentions, regularly journalling their own practice in order to value, analyse and change it appropriately. They are independent thinkers who act responsibly and develop effective strategies of accountability to their patients, colleagues and to the administration. They consistently read current journals, engage in nursing research and mentor new colleagues. They have highly developed interpersonal skills, a commitment to nursing as a profession, a sound, current knowledge of their nursing specialty and excellent clinical skills.

Perhaps you can see why I have identified the professional nurse as a mythical creature or a nursing educator's dream?

Demythologising nursing

The myth of the professional nurse exposes nursing education's philosophical commitments to the future of nurses and nursing. It is the language of nursing myth makers creating a new cultural myth of what it means to be a nurse in our eurocentric culture. However this process is constantly undermined by the prevailing power of the traditional nursing myth, subtly enacted and replicated through the daily rituals of nursing practice and through the embodied experiences of nurses. Peggy Chinn clarifies this when she challenges us to recognise that myths:

> are not entirely false and in fact contain an element of reality. This is why they are seductive and difficult to recognise. Since myths are based on a particular world view, they function actually to shape and create reality. Until we examine myths critically, we are not able to sort what is ill founded from that which is well founded, or whose interests are served (Chinn 1985:45).

This plea for a critical analysis of the myths which govern our lives is particularly pertinent for nursing. Nursing myths are created from images and symbols which are historically embedded in the commonsense knowledge of what it means to nurse, and they are lived out daily through the process of embodiment in nursing practices.

Chinn (1985) is wisely suggesting that through the process of laying myths open to analysis we can recognise both the destructive and constructive elements inherent in them. This is a significant movement away from a rationalist assumption that myths belong to the realm of the pre-scientific, and that mythical thinking can be purged from our culture. Indeed belief in a capacity to live rationally uninfluenced by the power of myth is one of the most powerful myths of our age. Its power lies in its assumption that we can be totally rational people unaffected by our cultural heritage, our personal history, our psycho-social needs for security, for acceptance, and for nurturance. It also assumes a link between rationality and happiness, which I contend, along with Fay (1987), is impossible to substantiate because we are not disembodied and culture-free. We are embodied, culturally embedded and relational beings, who are subject to inconsistencies and influences. Our lives are not rational. We are influenced by mythical thinking, by aesthetics, by spirituality, by tradition, by rituals and by culturally created habitual ways of experiencing the world around us.

Demystifying the feminist journey with nursing

A brief analysis of the progress of the women's movement in demystifying 'woman' from the 1960s and 1970s (see Friedan 1963, Greer 1970, de Beauvoir 1961) can be instructive in demonstrating the power of myth in our lives. The work of the feminists in the sixties and seventies focused on identifying and owning a critique of the ideological construction of woman as a creature of myth, created and sustained by patriarchy. This process of demystification required systematic rational and analytical thought to identify and repudiate the images and metaphors inherent in the symbolic concept of 'woman' formed through, and serving the interests of, patriarchy.

This patriarchal myth of woman was systematically dismantled and the rhetoric of the liberal feminists suggested that the emergent woman had discarded the myths of womanhood for the reality of rationality. The identity of woman became a cultural site of struggle exposing contradictory forces, points of fragility, and examples of accommodation and resistance, as women, along with some male colleagues, attempted to understand and rationally reclaim women from patriarchy (e.g. Harding 1986). This was mirrored in the energetic way nursing leaders conspired to compete with doctors and administrators in their own territories without demythologising the bases of these territories. It was demonstrated in an un-questioning adoption of the scientific method where people were reduced to systems. It was evident in nursing management theories which turned ill people into inputs, throughputs and outputs without adjusting funding formulas to account for human diversity. This liberal feminist approach was also evident in the push for autonomy in nursing practice. It was best exemplified in the increasing autonomy of community health nurses, community midwives and private practice nurses. These nurses benefited from the liberal feminist demands for autonomy and parity. However the majority of nurses working in institutional contexts were required to work with patriarchally constructed medical teams and were unable to act in ways which were equitable and autonomous.

In contrast to the liberal call for equity and autonomy, critical social scientists were challenging women in health care to become 'engaged' so as to make their world rational and just (Fay 1977). This carried an inherent assumption that women could suddenly live lives that were rational and just merely by undertaking an intellectual commitment. That kind of thinking denies the power of embodied rituals and traditions in our lives. In attempting to live out this assumption women began to discover that 'rational and just' did not always equate to happiness or valuing other capacities such as nurturance, awareness, consensus or holism (Street 1992).

In response radical feminists, such as Daly (1978), Raymond (1986), and Christ and Plaskow (1979) led the way for a rediscovery, recovery and redefinition of the 'essential woman' gleaned from examinations of matriarchal cultures. This is a form of regenerative myth making and the genesis of a new mythology about women which is supported by both newly created and re-emergent rituals. Nurses interested in this approach worked together to develop communities where new rituals which honored women and nursing incorporated women's rituals and knowledge from the past (Wheeler & Chinn 1989).

However often the feminist concern with changing the situation for women presupposed an 'essential' woman, who was inevitably white, middle class, educated, eurocentric and heterosexual. This 'essential' woman, whose experience could be implied to be similar for all women, earned critique from feminists who are women of color (e.g. hooks 1981, Hull, Scott & Smith 1982), women from developing countries (e.g. Spivak 1990, Minh-ha 1991) and lesbians (e.g. Frye 1992, Lorde 1984, Johnston 1973). Each has challenged the myth of the essential women from their own standpoint.

As Spivak commented:

> I am dubious about the present trend of speaking about the cultural construction of gender and race...It should also be said in these high-minded arguments about the cultural construction of gender and race, implicitly, the heterogeneity of one's own culture is protected, because one sees oneself as outside of the cultural construction of gender and race or as a victim of it; whereas the homogeneity of other cultures is implicitly taken for granted...you don't in fact talk about your own culture at all, although you do talk about other cultures as if they were homogeneous (1990:123).

Many nurses are understandably suspicious of the categorising of feminists. They share concerns that their experiences were not represented in the language and expectations held by society in relation to the term 'feminist'. Nancy Fraser and Linda Nicholson (1988) challenge the notions of any totalising positions such as a 'feminist standpoint', 'a women's perspective'; or 'the root cause of women's oppressions'. They contend that if the universalisms of humanity are suspect then so also must be the universalisms of gender. Gunew (1990) agrees and argues:

What feminist theorists need to reiterate with wearisome regularity is the diversity and specificity of women rather than any notional woman (Gunew 1990:29).

In the same way we need to reiterate with wearisome regularity the diversity and specificity of nurses rather than the notion of a generalised person who is a nurse. According to one clinical nurse:

There's such a very wide range commitment in intelligence, of capability, of ideology and all that sort of stuff that makes it so difficult to work out what exactly nursing is and why people do it and what they want out of it.

The myth that nurses do not have a distinct nursing culture is to be resisted, but also to be resisted is the notion that all nurses are the same—that a nurse is a nurse is a nurse.

TRANSCULTURAL MYTHS

Nursing is beginning to also take seriously the issues of ethnicity, and the movement in transcultural nursing, led by Madeleine Leineinger (1988) is a demonstration of this. The serious and sensitive work done by Thompson (1991) typifies thoughtful cultural work. Our own work with nurses examining the issues involved in caring for ill children and families from non English speaking backgrounds has found that many nurses are recognising the need to think seriously about the care for and the categorising of other ethnic groups (Parsons et al 1994). By placing the person from a different ethnic background as 'other' to themselves these nurses began to understand the process of 'othering the other'.

Effective communication is central to expert nursing practice. Communication issues are raised continually in discussions with clinical nurses concerning the frustrations and limitations of the nursing role. This is true when nurse and client share the same language, culture and social and economic positioning in society. When expert nurses find themselves limited by language and cultural barriers, the situation is more problematic. This is evident in some of the comments raised in the preliminary stages of a research project which worked with nurses to explore the issues inherent in their practice of caring for children and families from non English speaking backgrounds (NESB). As the nursing staff considered their practice it was evident that at all stages of the passage of the ill child and family, from the home, through the hospital visit and back into the community, ineffective communication created huge problems for the nurse and the family. Communication is always a concern of hospital staff with people from English speaking backgrounds, who are required to come to terms with medical jargon and hospital institutional practices. For families from non English speaking backgrounds the potential for difficulties is compounded on all sides. Ineffective communication may lead to people finding themselves the victims of labelling, stereotyping and being regarded as 'special needs' clients.

During the research process, nursing staff became aware that they only called upon interpreters for doctors or social workers. They did not regard their own need to communicate with families as important as the need for doctors to give medical information. As one nurse said:

Isn't it interesting that we don't value our own work enough to think it is worth while to get an interpreter to do our bit, but as soon as a doctor has got something to say we all say, 'Oh, we'll get an interpreter'. It is sad really.

Communication issues add stress to nurses and patients alike, as is evident in the experience one nurse recounted:

Look this family from Peru has arrived with nothing...no clothes, no toothbrush, no comb, no letters from the referring doctor, no Medicare card, just nothing and they don't seem to want us to touch the child...I don't know if they know what is going to happen and I can't find out if she has been fasted, and the doctor hasn't arrived to get the interpreter, and we need a signed consent form.

Another nurse reflected in her journal on her experience of walking through the waiting room of the emergency department of the hospital and noticing that about 80% of the families there were very obviously from a non English speaking background. This nurse considered the effect of the normalising practices of the triage system for the people who arrive on the doorstep of a hospital in a busy multicultural city:

Just looking at them sitting around I wondered what they were thinking; did they understand the system? Did they feel able to ask the nurses if they wanted anything? Did they realise that their child had been assessed by a nurse and that this assessment had allocated them to an area of care? Had they been able to tell the nurse the real problems affecting the child and/or the family?

She continued to explore questions relating to the habitual taken for granted practices of the busy nurses working in the hustle and bustle of the place:

Had the nurses felt that they had ascertained the true problems? Had the nurses been interested in trying to? Had an interpreter been readily available would it have made the assessment easier? I know from past experience that nurses often hold off calling an interpreter for the nursing assessment as they will have to come again when the doctor wants to see the family. In these cases the assessment reverts to an objective assessment only and many issues identified in a subjective assessment may be missed.

This nurse is questioning the belief that all people who present at the hospital door are given the same standard of quality care. The medical care may be the same if an appropriate diagnosis his made. However how does the nurse provide for the social and emotional care of frightened families with ill babies when there is no real understanding of the specific needs of the family? The reassuring conversation so crucial in crisis situations is not possible.

Nurses who have come to Australia from non-western countries, speak of the denial of their different knowledge and expertise and the effect of this on the people in their care. As one nurse explained:

My country Malaysia is a country with many cultures, many different religions, different traditions. My family is Buddhist but I trained in a hospital where we had many Muslim women coming, and they would only want the women doctors and women nurses to look after them. They can't have a man who is not their husband see their bodies. We all know this and we make the arrangements. So when I saw this Muslim woman come in and be sat in the queue for Dr A then I knew we would have trouble. Dr A is a good doctor but the Muslim woman...She can't undress in front of a strange man. I looked on the list and there were only men doctors here today, and so I spoke to the charge nurse and she said, 'Well we can't do anything, she'll just have to see Dr A'. I spoke to the woman and explained. She really looked very ill by now and was obviously in great pain, and had left it as long as she could before coming in, and she was with her daughter. I was very concerned for her and tried to find a doctor from another area to look at her as she needed to be admitted but I got nowhere. People were sympathetic but no one did anything. They just said that she would have to see Dr A and of course when she went in she refused to let him touch her. He had a nurse in there but she wasn't going to let a strange man see her parts and she just refused and we were all frustrated, but she got in the taxi and went home in agony. I felt so helpless and wished people had taken my concerns more seriously. Many Australians think that because something is all right for them then it has to be all right for everyone who lives here. It's not like that. People don't just give up their own ways because they live in another country. I often wondered what happened to her.

This story demonstrates the difficulty for everyone when a system is unable to meet needs of a minority group in the community.

THE MYTH OF HETEROSEXUALITY

Another common myth is that all nurses and their patients are heterosexual. Homosexual men and lesbian women are strongly represented in the community and in nursing as a discipline. Generally the homosexual men are well treated and accepted by the mainly female nursing population. However lesbian feminism is rarely discussed as a feminist category at nursing conferences or in nursing feminist papers, a recent paper by Hitchcock and Wilson (1992) being one of the few exceptions. The propensity of feminist nurses to ignore lesbian feminism is a sign of the power of the patriarchal symbolic order. It is a form of boundary control which rejects the unsayable. The boundaries are drawn by feminist nurses eager to be seen to be articulating a safe feminism for nursing, one which will attract the majority of nurses but which ignores the number of nurses and their patients who are indeed lesbians and are constructing their own views of reality through their own discourses. Martin (1992) describes the situation for lesbians:

We're acceptable as long as we don't demand a visible place among normal folk...we are not always confronted with direct, coercive efforts to control what we do in bed, but we are constantly threatened with erasure from discursive fields where the naturalisation of sexual and gender norms works to obliterate actual pluralities (1992:95).

One lesbian nurse commented on this form of erasure and its effects as:

Lesbians are everywhere in the health service—as nurses, educators, social workers, administrators and medical staff. But you would hardly know it. In particular there is a lack of lesbian visibility in nursing. High profile nurses who are in educational or clinical areas are often closeted about their lesbianism. Its usually known, in the 'family' so to speak, about so and so living with so and so for years. But these nurses mix in strictly elite lesbian social circles, if they mix at all.

This nurse went on to argue that the effect of this closeted life led to a denial of the lesbian nurse as an ordinary person:

You would rarely see these lesbian nurses supporting local lesbian events. You would rarely see them walking hand in hand down the street. No discussions at morning tea about the lover's latest problem with the relatives or how the joint mortgage was going. I can't help but feel disappointment that these women are unable to talk and live freely about a big part of their lives, their lovers, their sexuality. We shouldn't have to protect ourselves all the time from living and life.

The perpetuation of the myth that all nurses are heterosexual means that gay and lesbian nurses are not able to speak about their lives in normal ways. This form of silencing maintains the hegemony of heterosexuality which can have repercussions for the individual nurse, his or her peers and the people in their care.

As one gay nurse commented:

This lack of gay and lesbian visibility at the management level filters down to nursing at all other levels. But what it means is that if others don't know that we are caring professional nurses, who happen to be gay or lesbian, then our patients and clients who are gay or lesbian won't get the understanding they need.

A recent article in *Paediatric Nursing* argues that lesbian and gay parents are the hidden group of parents whom paediatric nurses need to acknowledge and whose lifestyle they need to understand (Rose 1993:199). Rose argues that it has been well documented that nurses tend to have rigid and conservative attitudes about sexuality which affect their behavior to same-sex families.

Both lesbian and heterosexual nurses have spoken to me of their concern that lesbian couples were not given the same rights as male/ female couples when they had a child in hospital. As one nurse explained:

If a woman has a man with her and they act as if they are together then we don't ask them if they are married or anything. We accept that they are a couple and may want to stay together to support each other. But I noticed that the other day, when a woman wanted to stay overnight with her (female) partner to support her when their child was hospitalised, the nurse told them, 'Only the parent can sleep' and they said 'We are both her parents' and she said, 'Well only one of you can stay'. This nurse told me this at handover, and I asked her why she hadn't let them both stay as they were the parents of the child, and she said, 'Well I can't cope with that'. I mean this baby was really sick and the woman needed her partner and her partner was worried sick and kept phoning. It was just discrimination.

Many same-sex couples censor themselves out of fear that the hospital staff will not understand and support their situation. As Rose (1993) reminds us:

> A major part of the paediatric nurse's role is to involve families in the care of their child by ensuring that parents are kept fully informed of the child's condition and progress. If the parents are pretending to be 'just good friends' then one or the other will not have equal access to information about their child (p. 19).

Another lesbian nurse reported that when her partner went to hospital the staff would only give information to her 'immediate family' which they considered was her mother who phoned from interstate. The ill woman hadn't seen her mother for four years but her need to be with her partner of the past six years was ignored by the staff, causing anguish to both of them.

The reports of the struggles of gay men to legitimate their right to spend time with their partners dying from AIDS has been well documented in the media and in books (Foster 1993). Equally, other same sex partnerships are often invisible in a health system when they are most vulnerable.

THE MYTHICAL PRE-EMINENCE
OF MEDICAL RESEARCH

Recent gains in remuneration and conditions for nurses coupled with an increasingly technical role have persuaded some clinicians and nurse scholars that medical domination and oppression by gender are no longer key issues for nurses. The more obvious manifestations of these forms of hierarchically formed oppression have indeed begun to disappear from our hospital units. We no longer see nurses stand when a doctor enters a room, and many nurses are feeling increasingly comfortable about challenging medical incompetence and ignorance when they meet it in their daily work. However a closer examination of the power relationships in clinical and research activities demonstrates that the myth of medical dominance is alive and well.

There has been much talk about the problem of doctors using nurses as data collectors for their research projects but little has been done to challenge this widespread practice. Unit managers give permission for nurses to be involved as they see the benefits for the patients and accept the doctor's assurances that the work can be incorporated into nursing practice. So, instead of applying for funding to employ nurses as data collectors, doctors continue to use nurses as unpaid labor and through this process limit even further the capacity of nurses to engage in their own research. The effect of this was evident in the following reflection from one nurse who wanted some free time to do a literature search for her participatory research group:

I was actually getting a little frustrated the other day. Our ward being a general medical ward, there are two medical research projects going on at the moment, and I was getting a little bit frustrated in the staff meeting the other day. Both doctors have spoken to us separately and we actually have a little bit more of a workload because of this, and that's fine. We have to take bloods, 'cos the blood sisters won't take them, and I mean they've got their reasons for it, but that means that we have to take pre and post medication levels on two occasions really. There's just extra work for us. And I was just sort of sitting there thinking, 'Well what about if I wanted to go down the library for half an hour?' Would the doctors be supportive of the fact that I wanted to go and do this? You know if it's all right for them to all say 'you know you've got to do this or that' and I thought, 'Well what about us?' I'm not just a little maid sitting on the ward doing everything. So I was getting a little bit frustrated thinking, 'Well I feel as if they're gaining something out of their work and they're learning something, but sometimes I feel that if I come to work, do my work, go home, don't have time for anything else. By the time I get home I just feel exhausted, where a day (release for research) would be fantastic' (Street & Walsh 1994a).

It is interesting to see this nurse beginning to unpick the myth of the pre-eminence of medical research. Although at the start of the conversation she says that it is 'fine' for the doctors from two research projects to use her as a data collector, she then spends the rest of the time explaining how she is beginning to understand that it is not 'fine'. She provides a picture of herself as a nurse who wants to spend time in the library investigating the topic of interest to herself and her colleagues rather than being a little maid sitting on the ward awaiting the doctor's orders. In this account she demonstrates her capacity to demythologise the prevailing belief and to begin to remythologise her own script.

CONTROL MYTHS

The women's movement continues to engage in the task of demythologising and remythologising woman against a backdrop of patriarchal culture. This same project of demythologising and remythologising is a seminal task for nursing. This implies that nursing needs to engage in a similar struggle to unlearn and unthink the old ways of being nurses and knowing nursing. This process begins with the process of identifying that traditional nursing myths are not in tatters as we would want to believe. I would like to suggest that we have become so familiar with the critique of common elements of these traditional myths, and of the remarkable recent gains which nurses have won for themselves, their patients and the health of the community at large, that we often ignore the perpetuation of these old ideas in new and subtle forms.

We fail to comprehend fully that the potency of the traditional myth to control nursing action is disguised but not diminished. The role of 'control myths' in the lives of women has been expounded by Lipman-Blumen (1984), who identifies the ways in which women have been controlled by the myths of patriarchy. These myths deceive by appearing to assign desirable characteristics to woman such as selflessness, thereby locking them into ongoing altruism in an uneven race with the men of patriarchal societies who are freed from this obligatory social virtue and can single mindedly pursue their own ends. Nurses and nurse scholars can benefit from an examination of the ways in which control myths are present in nursing practice and in curriculum initiatives.

The power of these control myths in nursing can be discovered as nurses examine the dilemmas and contradictions inherent in their clinical and curriculum practices. According to Foucault (1977), power is not exercised hierarchically, but through a complex web of structures and relationships. This is a helpful insight as we work together to uncover the web of power relations associated with control myths in nursing.

In order to counter the power of control myths, Rowland (1988) encourages women to engage in the power of disbelief. I find such skepticism is an essential underpinning to participatory research because it enables us to negate illusory and limiting myths and affirm stories and symbols that are restorative.

An understanding of the presence of, and processes by which nurses take part in, rituals born of mythical thinking can enable nurse educators to develop curriculum processes that facilitate critical reflection in nurses. Nurses meeting together in PAR groups at the Royal Children's Hospital are working to make creative spaces where nurses can meet and share accounts of their practice, analyse the values and implications inherent in them, develop strategic plans for change, implement the changes and reflect together on the experience in order to understand and plan future action. Through the process of acceptance, mutual support and a lot of laughter and tears nurses can begin to unlearn defensiveness and learn to challenge with authenticity and integrity. Together nurses are discovering the power to disbelieve the control myths that disempower nurses and patients.

Control myths are sustained through language practices, moral judgements and value stances which are often unexpressed and unacknowledged. We are discovering the subtleties of disempowering language as we hear ourselves speak in the group. We hear ourselves say:

No, he is not a doctor. He is just a nurse!

It is the job of the primary nurse to ask the doctor what he wants done with his patient.

Let's ask the girls if they want to change the format for the nursing care plans.

As we talk together in the group we find out how to identify and unlearn disempowering habitual language patterns. An understanding of the complexities of habitual patterns can help nurses elucidate the cultural construction of nursing. Sophisticated analyses of nursing can then be created. These analyses will account for competing discourses while demonstrating an awareness of the dangers of developing totalising, elitist, racist and reductionist theories of nursing practice.

Collaborating together in this way is to take seriously the contention that as women have been colonised by men, so nurses have been colonised by the dominance of the medical discourse. As McLaren and Hammer remind us:

Colonial characteristics do not inhere in the genes...they are learned. False histories, false role models, and false expressions of a people's creative potential together with socially imposed constraints that perpetuate these false belief systems keep the colonised in place...in other words, the colonised are taught to believe the dominant ideological myths about their collective being, and act accordingly (1989:45).

The challenge for nurses is to discover the many myths masquerading in the discourses of patriarchy and medicine. These nursing myths encapsulate false histories, false role models and the false expectations of people's capacity to heal. Nurses need to rediscover that healing can occur in many ways: ways which may be innovative; ways which may be traditional; and ways which may blend the old and the new to heal body, mind, spirit and the earth.

Another task of demythologising is to identify moral judgements which affect the ways that nurses work and interact with patients and colleagues. These judgements become transparent when nurses are prepared to acknowledge their own taken for granted values and to think about how they impinge upon their judgements and actions towards others whose values are different. Challenges to moral judgements enable nurses to become sensitive to remarks such as:

I didn't have any trouble orienting this new nurse because she was hospital trained and so knew how to work properly.

I don't care if that mother is overtired. She shouldn't take out her anger on the nursing staff. We are all going to refuse to look after her daughter if she is transferred back here.

Listening to our comments or examining our values in action, we begin to uncover the ways in which our practices are entrenched in culturally created, habitual attitudes and disempowering language. We find that the values which we hold dear are not always apparent in our practices; indeed we regularly discover that our actions represent values which we may believe we have discarded.

REMYTHOLOGISING NURSING MYTHS

The philosophy of a paediatric hospital is shaped around rhetoric that the interests of the child and the family are paramount. A gulf between rhetoric and reality is present in this and any other hospital. However, the role that everyday nursing rituals and practice play in the perpetuation of rhetoric and myth that are not necessarily of the nurses' own making is not always immediately apparent.

Until fairly recently it has been widely asserted by the medical profession that young children don't experience pain with the same intensity as adults. This myth has enabled medical staff to engage in painful procedures on young children without the complications of analgesia and anaesthetic. However, the nurses who care for these young children have observed that they do in fact feel pain, and have suffered feelings of guilt and anguish in participating in painful procedures. In order to continue to work in units where children routinely experience painful procedures nursing staff learn various de-sensitising myths such as: 'Small children don't feel pain', 'Everyone gets hurt in life they just have to learn to cope' and the most disempowering one:

> I hate hurting children but they have to have these painful procedures and I can't change anything.

In response to these myths, we decided to spend time making careful and detailed observations of the children's reactions during painful procedures in order to understand something of what it was like for them. The first observation was carried out by a nurse and myself as we watched a wriggling child having her coronal traction re-bandaged by a colleague prior to surgery. Although we were focusing on the experience of a 13 month old child, three things became apparent to us. We could call them three myths in action.

The first myth in action we noticed was that halfway through the procedure when the child gave up struggling and lay still she had not succumbed to the charm of the nurses, and neither was she pain-free: she was in a state described by the nurse as despair. The nurse observing with me noticed this and said:

> So that's what they mean in the literature about despair. I've known about it but I have never seen it. I guess I didn't want to.

Although this nurse had read in the literature about despair in children as an effect of institutionalisation, she recognised that in reality she and her colleagues often worked as if children did not despair. They convinced themselves that their efforts had made a difference because they were not carefully observing the effects of their actions on those receiving their care.

The second myth in action we uncovered was that when nurses are working together they are working as a functional team. The language nurses use such as, 'Will you help me remove this chest drain?' carries no further detailed discussion. The assumption is that nurses are clear about how to carry out their role in the team. Our observations showed that rather than functioning smoothly and efficiently the nurses often competed to do parts of the task and relate to the child. They interrupted each other's interactions and cut across each other's roles during the procedure. This could be expected as these nurses do not regularly carry out this procedure together. Yet the lack of teamwork was not immediately apparent to the nurses concerned who felt that the procedure went reasonably well. It was only through discussion of the effect of the procedure on the child that we were able to discover the results of a subscribing to a mythical idea about holistic care This myth suggested that it should be possible for any single nurse to give total care by conducting a complex and painful procedure on an active toddler while at the same time meeting the emotional needs of the parent and the child. The taken for granted assumption was that an effective team could be formed by bringing together any nurses who knew what was required in terms of the procedure and the psycho-social needs of the child and parents.

The third myth in action concerned the changes of the emotional state of the child depending on whether the parent's attention was focused on her child or with the staff. There is nothing new or surprising about this, and yet the nursing staff's concept of keeping the patient and family informed meant that they kept explaining things to the mother as the procedure went along. The child showed further distress, and the nurses would vie with the parent to distract and amuse the child.

During the observation of the rebandaging of the child's traction, the parent was seated behind the child's head. She was not in a good position to engage freely with her child, nevertheless the child kept twisting her body back towards her mother, something which made the work of the nurses harder. In this instance the whole procedure took twenty-three minutes with everyone feeling glad it was over. We discussed the experience and after locating these difficulties deliberately set out to change the situation for the child and the parent on the following day. To do this we took some basic principles as the basis for the reconstructed action.

We decided to make the child's comfort the main focus. We recognised that small children do give up in despair when they have repeated experiences of pain. We also acknowledged that quietness does not always mean that they have been comforted by the nurse saying 'It's nearly finished, nearly finished' when the procedure is not nearly finished at all. Nor do children necessarily concur with the nurse's 'It doesn't hurt now' when what is happening is still painful or frightening. The nurses talked about hearing themselves and their colleagues reassure their patients inappropriately because they themselves were under stress and wished that the procedure was painless, comfortable and could be finished quickly.

Through discussion the nurses recognised that the development
of effective teamwork required communication and negotiation,
no matter how temporary the team was to be, as is the case with a
single procedure. They found that a team could function well if
each person took a particular role in the team and did not attempt
to carry out all the competing roles concurrently. Effective
communication with the relative or friend of the patient meant
that they could participate as members of the temporary team
allowing the patient to be distracted or comforted by someone who
knew them well and understood their specific needs. This required
the nurses to brief the relative or friend on the effects of the
procedure and the role of distracting the patient. The nurses could
continue with the technical aspects of the procedure while not
interrupting their colleagues or, more importantly, the interaction
between the relative and the patient. Observations of the nursing
practice based on these simple principles showed that the task would
be less uncomfortable for the patient, would be done more quickly,
would require fewer staff and cause less disruption to routines.

As these nurses met regularly in participatory research groups
and experienced the value of the support of colleagues they began
to understand how the lack of collegiality had affected the care
they provided and the relationships they formed with their peers.
They were able to see that the mythical nursing team was often not
a functioning reality. Nurses confessed that they would often go
home feeling unfulfilled and guilty because they had not been able
to provide the kind of care that they expected of themselves and
others and that this guilt often led to 'horizontal violence' (Freire
1972). As one nurse reported:

Yeah, no, we don't support each other. I was just saying like we did
this study in my honors year on horizontal violence in nursing, and I
think that it's atrocious, and I think that we're all our own worst enemies.
No one ever says, 'You've done a fantastic job on that today'. They're
the first to point out if something's gone wrong. I really think that it's
because we all feel so oppressed within the institutions.

Other nurses argued that the participatory nature of the research
processes enabled them to discover different ways to work together
and to understand how supportive processes work. As one nurse
commented:

I'm not quite sure what it is, but I think that we're a really disbanded
body of people, and I think that if we're ever going to change nursing,
and sort of move ourselves up...that we've got to work together, as

opposed to working against each other, which, I think is, what's happening on general things. Not just the ward environment, but from the hierarchy. I feel that the hierarchy don't really don't support the ward nurses enough. And I feel that the ward nurses don't support each other enough. So I certainly think that working together [is] a clue to our movement forward. They don't support what you're doing; they don't see the value in what you're doing. People have to come to an understanding that we have to work together to improve the ward. Support means not just talk. It means senior nurses taking on more patients for half an hour while you have your research meetings. That's what it means! I certainly think our culture does preclude that. I don't know how we're ever going to get over that, I really don't.

This nurse is putting her finger on the difference between the rhetoric of support for research with its practical reality—rearranged priorities and action taken to facilitate research activities.

It is through discussion and analysis of control myths which construct the world of nursing practice that it becomes possible to renounce them and the rituals through which they are enacted. It is a process of disbelieving the myths. For example, in the interests of patients, nurses can take to themselves the power to disbelieve the tenet of nursing administration that all nurses are adaptable to any context—a control myth which enables nursing administrators to move nurses from one specialist practice to another like chess pieces to cope with shortages. I recognise that this is a provocative statement which flies in the face of the assumptions of nursing education and administrative practices and so I want to emphasise here that I am not talking about student nurses or novices. The implications of Benner's (1984) study of novice to expert demonstrated that this myth of the ever adaptable nurse is a project in deskilling because it does not allow nurses to develop into expert practitioners. In their action research project, East and Robinson (1994:60) found that the problem of 'keeping up the numbers' meant that nurses were considered 'virtually interchangeable'—a continued process of deskilling.

This deskilling process becomes more apparent when we think about the systematic and structured skilling of medical staff. Although medical students, interns and residents have a comprehensive introduction to a range of medical specialties, no cardiac surgeon is ever moved to the ophthalmology unit for a session because there is a vacancy, and no physician is ever drafted to do a spot of neurosurgery for a day. We may then like to ask ourselves why cardiac specialist nurses can be sent to general medical units or oncology nurses sent to general surgical units? Whose interests are being served by the retention of these practices? We cannot lay all the blame on the structures which maintain this practice of 'sending' nurses to help out in other specialties. We begin to recognise that nursing administrators often are forced to make these decisions 'in the interests of patient care' because nurses themselves are so mobile. The tourist nurse is alive and well with a 'ticket to ride', flitting around the hospitals of the world and leaving vacancies to be filled by another nurse from any place nursing administration can find them. Unfortunately such mobility also means that nurses leave one ward, or one hospital, for another when they feel powerless to effect change, thereby perpetuating the view of the nurse as ever adaptable, and ever powerless. The term 'multi-skilling' has been coined and is being loosely applied to defend the movement of staff from one place to another without examining the need to be skilled effectively before multi-skilling is a possibility. This is not only an issue for groups of nurses in hospitals or for administrators or for educators, but an issue for the whole discipline.

In participatory research groups we began to question the entrenched idea that we have no responsibility for the resources of the earth. Nurses are beginning to appreciate the link between their practice and a vision of the natural splendor and power of the world in which they live, of regions yet to be destroyed at the hand of rational, scientific and technological humanity. Feminist nurses such as Helen Lucas of 'Nursing the Environment', who incidentally wants 'to save the earth before lunch', have taken seriously the concern that nurses care enough to heal the earth. For example, nurses do need to analyse and challenge the myths of cleanliness which result in practices of using and misusing unrenewable resources and work to raise the awareness of others in the hospital. However, key support for nurse environmentalists from members of the health field has mostly come in the areas of waste management and recycling as these are the areas of cost savings—the interests of the economists and the administrators. Although these issues are important, other feminist nurses such as Martin (1990) are concerned to explicate the links between modern and traditional healing knowledge and practices and the rhythms of the earth and of life.

It is important to affirm that the power to disbelieve control myths is developed collaboratively. Through discussion nurses have noted that they have been powerfully and profoundly inculcated into the desirability of ceaseless activity. As embodied beings they have become aware that ceaseless activity is inscribed upon the sinews and muscles of their bodies in ways that make them uneasy and restless when they are not being busy bees. They have learnt only to feel good about themselves when they have concrete proof of their activities. When the day stretches behind full of tangible tasks which are obvious to all then they can *feel* confident, but when the day appears to have been spent in activities which are not readily apparent, feelings of confidence can plunge. When nurses make reasoned decisions to cultivate reflective processes regularly they discover the limitations laid upon them by this historically and culturally created embodiment. The decision to keep a journal of clinical or teaching practice, or make a priority of forming or regularly attending a group aimed at reflection, ideology-critique and empowering praxis, recedes under the compulsion of their bodies to engage in constant movement. To change the rituals of ceaseless activity requires the development of a disbelief in the control myth of nurses as 'doers'. It means rejecting physical reactions which enslave in habitual, ritualised ways of being. This process of active disbelieving is a very difficult process of unlearning. And it is it very hard, if not impossible, to unthink and unlearn in isolation. Meeting together regularly to encourage each other in the project of unlearning constant busyness and following reflective processes has led some nurses to change.

However the process of setting up participatory research groups has required the power to undo the myth that the modern nurse has no time for writing, talking, researching or reflecting on clinical practice. Collaborative reflection helps isolate the disempowering potential of rituals that nurses subscribe to.

An examination of a seemingly insignificant ritual in a large adult public hospital in Melbourne is tying back the curtains around beds with a careful bow. Of course this bow has to be untied and retied every time the curtains need to be pulled back or forward. A colleague and I have estimated that it takes about one minute to tie and untie the bow and that this would occur on an average of ten times each day for each patient. As a nurse on this ward is responsible for the care of six patients the ritual alone can take one hour per nurse per day. If we are talking about a 450 bed hospital with an average of 382 beds occupied daily on an occupancy rate of 80% we could be talking about 63 and a half hours of combined nursing staff time spent each day untying and retying bows. This is 11.7 effective full time per week of nursing time engaging in this ritual—without taking into account the times the bow is tied too tight, the patient desperately needs privacy, the bow has to be cut, and a new tie procured from the storeroom and pinned into place. The necessity for this, and similar rituals needs to be balanced against claims by nurses of insufficient time to think, talk and reflect on the care they provide for their patients.

The power released through collaboration, and a commitment to the best interests of their patients and to their colleagues, enables nurses not only to disbelieve the control myths of nursing but also enables them to believe in the potential of remythologising of nursing. They need to continue to disbelieve in control myths if they are to identify mythical elements in clinical practice. The other side of the power to demythologise is the power to remythologise, that is the power to believe; the power to reconstitute the myth of the professional nurse by believing and acting as if nurses can contribute to it becoming a reality. This entails the exercise of the power to believe in the capacity of nurses to create new rituals to replace the traditional ones of dependence and oppression. Creating life-affirming and enabling rituals is easier said than done but many nurses are beginning to make a difference for themselves, their colleagues and the wider community through the development of collaborative research groups. These groups not only encourage the evolvement of empowering praxis based on understanding and critique, but also take account of the feminist values of inter-relationship, nurturance, passion and intuition. The restructuring of transformative rituals is mirrored in empowering and enabling nursing myths which speak of the place of health and illness and demonstrate ways to join together in the development of nursing.

2. Being caring: getting beyond the tyranny of niceness

Caring, then, even when performed with love, is frequently laborious and stressful. It is a highly charged emotional activity, where a carer's affective positioning can affect the quality of care that person is able to offer (Opie 1992:190).

Caring is a key concept for nursing. The literature is replete with discussions on the nature and purpose of caring in nursing culture (see Morse et al 1991 for a summary of all the theorists of caring). It is an area well canvassed by nursing academics (e.g. Benner & Wrubel 1989, Dunlop 1986, Kitson 1987, Leineinger 1984, 1988, Watson 1985, 1987, Walker 1993). Caring is a central part of nursing curricula.

During my doctoral study, I investigated an aspect of caring as the phenomenon of nurturance/knowledge (Street 1992a). When I began work as a researcher in a hospital I expected that caring would be a paramount concern to clinical nurses. I expected to find that caring would be a word on the lips of nurses and a word apparent in their documentation.

THE CARING UNIT

My initial discussions with clinical staff did not confirm the impression until I entered a particular unit for the first time and was greeted by the unit manager:

Welcome to the unit. I'm sure you will like working with us here; everyone does. It's a really caring unit. Everyone's so nice and friendly.

The unit manager then went on to introduce me to other staff, and sure enough, they did seem nice and they did seem friendly, and I heard similar comments from staff such as:

Welcome to the unit. You will really like it here. Everyone is so caring. Everyone likes working here.

Oh this is a nice unit. Everyone's so friendly. We all socialise together; well some of us do anyway.

I am only new to this unit but already I've been invited to go out with a group of staff on Friday night. Everyone's so nice and friendly. It's a really caring unit.

To hear the same endorsements in essentially the same language from different staff within the space of two or three minutes was intriguing. My previous experiences of being introduced to other units had not included what almost amounted to a public relations exercise about how 'nice' and 'friendly' and 'caring' the nursing staff of the unit were. In fact it was so pervasive that it made me want to stop and find out what was really happening there. Did these nurses really have something special that they couldn't keep quiet about, or, was this a case of 'if we say this often enough we will all continue to believe it'? The nurses certainly looked happy and friendly as they flashed past me, rushing from one end of the unit to the other. They certainly seemed to have an excessive amount of 'thank you' cards and chocolates and flowers decorating the nurse's station. And when I listened to the conversations the word 'nice' seemed to be used regularly and it seemed to be used interchangeably with the word 'caring'.

I was perhaps sensitive to this point as the word 'nice' is one of those words which doesn't require any real commitment whereas the word 'caring' implies commitment and relationship, no matter how temporary the circumstances. I reflected upon this 'caring' unit and found myself thinking more generally about the concept of caring and nursing. I recognised myself as someone whose concept of care is more defined by what caring is not, rather than by what it is. In this sense, I realised I was representative of those clinical nurses whose understanding of caring is ill defined and replete with taken for granted assumptions.

Defining caring

When attempting to rectify this situation by re-reading some of the nursing theories that focus on the concept of caring, I began to incorporate all the different features which have been elucidated by various nursing theorists into the Annette Street all-purpose, all-embracing concept of caring. After considerable effort I managed to come up with a definition that only took up fourteen lines of typing. At this stage it occurred to me that my definition was beginning to be a trifle unwieldy:

*street
def of
caring*

Caring is a primary mode of being in the world, which is natural to us, and of significance in our relationships with others, which is evident in actions directed to assist, support or enable during those rare precious moments of unique encounter when the participants recognise this. Caring is the common base of humanity and so involves values, a will and commitment to care, knowledge, caring actions and consequences, attending to the 'objectness' of persons without reducing them to the moral status of objects but rather feeling dedication to another to the extent that it motivates and energises action to influence life constructively and positively, both by increasing intimacy and mutual self-actualisation. Caring exists when the nurse harmoniously demonstrates verbal caring, non-verbal caring and technically competent behaviour and focuses on the attainment and maintenance of health, or a peaceful death.

This definition turned out to be unhelpful except as something which enabled me to begin focusing on how complex the taken for granted concept of caring was. I decided that all-inclusive definitions had their limitations and I should abandon this to the nursing theorists.

Ignoring the Annette Street concise working definition of caring I began to think that we need to care about what we care for. That being caring requires us not only to care for others by attending to their particular, concrete, physical, spiritual, intellectual, psychic, and emotional needs, but also to care about the groups, environments and situations in which this caring for others occurs. As members of a global community this involves caring about the physical environment and the social, economic and political forces at work which create dehumanising conditions. In the health sector it means caring about the way that decisions are made in relation to the provision of health care, and how the power to make these decisions is exercised both at the macro level of government, institution and community and at the micro level of the nurse-person relationship. This means that nurses need to care about the kind of health service that is provided within which their relationships of caring for others are structured. An understanding of this macro-micro relationship enabled me to begin to work with clinical nurses to analyse what being caring means for them.

Unravelling the rhetoric of a caring unit

I want to reflect on the self-advertising caring unit that I described at the start of this chapter. I was invited to interview nursing staff of this unit about the changes to their roles since the introduction of a new clinical nursing career structure. I decided to conduct open ended interviews to enable the nurses to raise their own thoughts about the process. What emerged from the onset was the pervasive belief that the unit was a happy place where everyone was nice. However without exception each nurse interviewed claimed to be an outsider—someone who didn't really fit in with the rest of the unit. As I explored the reasons why they were claiming to be isolated from this apparently happy team I heard the same litany of concerns, which stemmed from a lack of significant relationship with others in the team. Relating at this shallow level meant that individual nurses felt unable to express their real concerns, their frustrations, their disappointments, their fears or their anger at the things they encountered in their daily work. As these feelings were not expressed in the work context they were not resolved creatively and individual nurses were blaming themselves for what were legitimate concerns. They all talked about taking home their frustrations at the things which made them feel powerless to provide effective care for seriously ill children. They discussed their self-recrimination, their feeling that they should have been able to do better in particular situations and in how they organised their work overall. Yet these were the same people who had all met at the pub for a good time after work, who claimed that everyone else was nice and caring and who were regarded as part of the 'in crowd' by the others.

As I listened to what these nurses were saying it became apparent that what they were experiencing was actually a form of oppression. They were negating their genuine experiences and feelings because they needed to fit into the unit stereotype of a 'nice, caring' person. They were being tyrannised by the unit culture and they were participating in policing their own oppression in a desire to be regarded as someone who is caring. In order to maintain the unit facade, individuals were not only acting in ways that were artificial but they were also setting up team relationships which fostered dependence rather than interdependence. As I considered this situation I labelled it the 'tyranny of niceness'. When I discussed this label with the nurses they knew immediately what I meant. They began to speak about how being caring is translated as 'being nice'; 'not making a fuss'; 'smiling a lot'; 'speaking in a sympathetic voice even if you go away and complain about the person afterwards'; 'not letting on that you think that the other person is being unfair'; and 'always putting the other person first even when you know they are a 'user''.

It seemed that the relationship between being nice and being caring had been blurred in such a way that these clinical nurses had subscribed to the notion that they were being genuinely caring when their commitment was to fit in with the unit expectations. Always appearing as a nice person served to distance them from constructive and creative caring relationships with those for whom they cared and with colleagues.

The tyranny of niceness

INTERESTING concept.

As I explored this concept of distancing I decided to investigate whether this unit was unique or whether other clinical nurses understood the label 'tyranny of niceness' as representing their own experience. I soon found that the 'tyranny of niceness' was a label which nurses could identify with regardless of whether they were located in the hospital, in community settings or in nursing academia.

As a nurse from another unit said:

Yes, that's it. You know I have thought about what happens to me when I feel angry about a situation and I do! Plenty of things happen here which are unfair and make me angry. But you see I know that I am expected to always stay calm. It's not considered nice to express your anger. We are children's nurses, we have to be nice people. When I listen to you talking about the 'tyranny of niceness' you are saying what I have felt but never really thought how to put into words. You just don't talk about those things. It's just not done.

In academic contexts nurse scholars reported their frustrations at the tyranny of niceness. Academics reported that they were expected to attend meetings where it was obvious that the decisions had already been made behind closed doors, and yet they were expected to maintain the facade that they were all in this together. As one academic commented.

A lot of energy at our place (university) goes into keeping things nice. We're all expected to be really positive about everything which gets dished up to us. We go to meetings and they are run like self-congratulatory exercises. Anyone who dares ask hard questions gets 'managed' by the executive group or frozen out. Yet there are many of us who would be prepared to be positive and contribute if we had a chance. There just doesn't seem to be a way to do it because we don't have access to the information, and to rock the boat is seen to be 'not nice'.

So for me the question became 'how does the tyranny of niceness affect the capacity of nurses to be genuine in their relationships and to make effective contributions in their situations?' If nurses are kept isolated from each other and from opportunities of admitting to their own feelings then it becomes difficult to get in touch with the feelings of others. This was particularly evident when I examined how care was provided. It was easy to see some superb individual instances of caring occurring every day on the units or in universities. Without a doubt nurses are people who do care deeply about their work and the people they care for. They do care for each other and for others in the health team. I personally experience and appreciate enabling care from the nursing staff and academics in the settings in which I work. However I also see and hear instances which demonstrate that nurses are subject to, and unwitting participants in, the tyranny of niceness. I was interested in exploring the concept further and the opportunity arose as I worked with different groups of nurses using participatory research processes.

Although the research questions of the participatory research groups vary greatly there are a number of concerns relating to nursing practice which emerge consistently for discussion regardless of the research topic. An examination of the nursing role and its relationship to the wider nursing culture is implicit in any research into clinical practice but in these participatory groups nursing role and nursing culture soon become explicit topics for conversation. However the counter culture nature of these participatory research processes mean they are often initially regarded with suspicion even by the clinical nurses who will benefit from them. It is only as we have worked together to unravel the situations which produce guilt in clinical nurses that they find themselves able to acknowledge they would like to be different. As a prelude to reconstructing attitudes and actions which are more genuinely caring, we have begun to understand those elements of nursing culture, those habits, attitudes and rituals which support the tyranny of niceness.

Researching a caring culture

Creating a research environment in a busy hospital is a counter culture activity in itself. Participation requires staff to reorganise their priorities and work practices to meet regularly, read, investigate, educate their peers, write about their clinical practice and evaluate their actions systematically and reflectively.

I will focus here on the work of one of these groups which was interested in examining a nursing practice with an empowering aim—to enable nurses to work with parents in determining how their children's care would be organised—but which caused the nurses some concern in its implementation.

Care by parent contracts

There are many daily activities that parents can do, or participate in, during their child's hospitalisation. This is good for the parent and good for the child. The parent feels connected and useful while the child knows familiar loving care in an unfamiliar, frightening environment. How this care is organised depends on the individuals. Whereas one mother may not want her child to associate her too strongly with hospital and leave the unpleasant activities to the nurses; another mother may feel that her child will trust her more than the nurse and she will know better how to handle and manage her own child.

The nurses working on the unit where the research took place, recognised the importance of parental involvement in the care of children and arranged for what are called 'care by parent' contracts. During admission, these contracts enable the nurses to sit down with the family members to discuss and document what involvement the family felt it would like to have in the care of the child during their stay in hospital. The aim of these contracts was to enable the parents or care givers to keep as much control as they wanted over the everyday activities such as feeding, washing or changing dressings. The nurses felt concerned that some parents started out taking on particular responsibilities but after a couple of days they would be less involved or disappear from the unit. The nurses also complained that some parents did not seem to take the contracts seriously.

The group then looked again at the small amount of literature on care by parent contracts. They found that these papers generally described what the contracts would involve and extolled their virtues, but that there was nothing written concerning the difficulties of implementation. The assumption was if you got the initial prescription right everyone would be happy.

The nurses then decided to collect more information about the care by parent arrangement by collecting stories from staff about the use of the contracts. This information showed that the nursing staff saw a contract as permanent rather than something that was open to constant negotiation every day or even every shift depending on the situation of the parent that day.

In order to get some feedback the staff arranged for me to speak to a few parents informally about what they thought about the care by parent contracts. The responses varied. Some parents reported feeling very happy to be involved, particularly fathers. They were bathing their children after work as they usually did at home instead of sitting helplessly by their children's beds in the unit. Others reported finding that they were getting very tired trying to cope with the hospitalised child while juggling their other family and work commitments. Some parents talked of the stress of being presented with a frightening diagnosis, and how coping with that had sapped their energy for the many care activities. So the nurses' initial concern was right—not all parents were experiencing the care by parent strategy as empowering. This was evident in new mother Rose's account of 10 week-old baby David's stay in hospital:

While his temperature was high, I didn't know what to do. I was really worried and suggested cool baths or boiled water and they (the nurses) said, 'If you want'…but I didn't have a clue—I hardly know how to look after a well baby, let alone a sick baby. In fact, I felt they left a lot up to me and wondered if they realised he was really sick and whether they were taking it seriously, but then I realised that they are probably used to heaps of desperately ill kids, but I'm not. Then I found a few days later by looking at David's folder that I was responsible for his general care, which I hadn't realised was the arrangement. I thought they had forgotten him…Another thing I was confused about, was how often the nurses and doctors would say, 'He's really looking great' or 'really well'…when I knew he'd had a high temperature in the night or something.

Rather than encouraging me, it made me feel that they didn't realise he was a sick boy.

I couldn't handle them telling me what I didn't feel was true. What was more comforting was when they looked worried about him. Then I knew they were really looking after him!

Rose went on to describe the nurses as 'really nice, really approachable'. Yet it is evident that these 'nice' nurses had not realised that although David was progressing well it was Rose who needed reassurance. The nursing staff were really surprised to hear Rose's side of the story because she was a popular parent on the unit and had been helpful to them at times when it was hectic. As we discussed this in a group, different nurses spoke of their frustrations with the heavy workload and the demands of the medical staff. They said that the need to 'nurse the doctor' prevented them from spending time with mothers like Rose who is warm, educated and appeared to be coping well with her son's hospitalisation. The nurses began to speculate that if Rose felt like this then they needed to understand the situation for other parents who appeared to have less support and fewer coping skills. This was a generic problem because often anxious parents were wanting to do everything they could when the child was admitted but as the days passed and the prognosis became clear, or the parent tired, their wish to be so involved changed. In Rose's case the admission process coincided with a time of high anxiety over David's condition. Although she had been taken through the care by parent contract by the admitting nurse, she had forgotten not only what she had agreed to do, but also that the contract even existed.

The nurses developed an action plan which involved spending time each shift reviewing the current situation with each parent finding out whether they still wanted to be involved in the care. The nurses wrote journal accounts to bring to the group meeting for analysis and reflection. As they explored this matter further they also recognised that if a parent was providing the basic care then it was important that nurses did not compete out of a concern that other staff might think them lazy. Nor was it appropriate to regard the care by parent arrangement as giving them more spare time. Rather they needed to regard the parents as the client and spend as much time with them as they would have on basic care for the child.

The term collaboration is often discussed in nursing literature but is not so evident on the units. We discovered that nurses saw themselves as team members whenever there was a physical task to be done but nurses would often not accept help when a particular parent required extra. The nurses considered that because they were rostered in charge of that particular family they should be able to handle any extra emotional demands. They stated that if they couldn't meet these demands they would regard themselves, and expect others to regard this, as a failure. This attitude had to be seen for what it was—rampant egotism masquerading under the label of autonomous nursing practice. It was evident in this, and in other similar situations, that interdependence was a better way for nurses to best care for these children, their families and nursing colleagues. The nurses in the group discovered that they were confusing individuality with the professional concept of clinical responsibility for the management of particular children. In the group we unpicked the way the concept of nursing autonomy had been distorted through the alienating practices of shift work, broken care and the patterns of avoidance. It appeared that isolated nurses developed avoidance behaviors to protect themselves when facing feelings of anger and frustration at watching children and families suffer. These nurses needed to care about each other in order to provide the best care for the seriously ill children in their charge.

Such reflections led to a change in the nurses' understanding and actions. They found that they were working as if the parents really were part of the health care team rather than the philosophy being just rhetoric and theoretical fantasy.

This is only one small example of how nurses work together in an endeavor to understand and restructure their clinical practices so as to care for the interests of the ill person and their family rather than responding to the competing demands of clinical rituals, or medical and administrative interests. These nurses were both courageous and supportive of each other as they put their clinical practices under scrutiny and began to discover that caring actions were actions which empowered people and that to do this required the restructuring of their workloads to prioritise time spent with people. The nurses in the group have been challenged to think about how they can collaborate to help each other meet the needs of the families in their care.

BEING CARING: REALLY COMMUNICATING

With another group of nurses engaging in a similar project we found that, although nurses would rehearse in their minds any new procedure, particularly one involving high technology, they would not rehearse how they might handle a parent who was particularly angry or upset or difficult. They relied upon an 'innate' capacity to care and communicate appropriately without recognising that genuine caring requires thought. We developed a much clearer understanding of those elements of nursing culture that dehumanise both care givers and receivers.

As we continued our investigations it became apparent to the nurses in the groups that, if their habitual, taken for granted practices and communication patterns weren't working well for English speaking families, they were much more problematic for children and families from non English speaking backgrounds. We decided that the tyranny of niceness was even more evident in the nursing provided to these families. Nurses reported that, as they didn't know how to communicate, they often coped with these families by smiling a lot and hurrying through the tasks.

The following discussion occurred during a research meeting. The group members were discussing the issue of what it would mean to be caring in a multicultural environment. Sharon began by saying:

Maybe we have to think about raising the awareness of the staff in taking the time to go through things more. Instead, it is very easy with those non English speaking parents for a staff member to whip through with the drug trolley, or when you are looking after the child to just give them a wash while mum sits by the bed and keeps the child company in their own language, and you don't spend the time with those people because you haven't got much to talk about. Maybe we need to spend that little bit of extra time, because they are the people that need the extra time, to 'sort of' explain things. Even if you have to wait for an interpreter, or if they have got a little bit of an understanding of English, to go through in very basic terms and diagrams and like getting the bottle and showing them...

Karen interjected:

Which means that we then have to address our own feelings about it, because you said we haven't got much to say to them, and we don't feel comfortable with them as much. We can't have that little chit chat.

Julie said:

You know yourself if someone with little English has said something to you twice and it is already twice, that you've said, 'I'm sorry can you repeat it', or, 'I don't understand', and they say that a third time and you say, 'Oh yeah', because you yourself are feeling embarrassed and inadequate. But you have not understood their attempt at English, so you can understand why they just nod first time round and say, 'Yes', with us, because it is just too hard for them to even try. I did it with Chang's mother the other day...Chang has been in and out of the unit, he is long term and I felt awful doing it to his mother...but it was up to the third or fourth time that I had asked her to repeat herself, and I thought I just can't do it again. I walked away and felt awful. She won't ask next time because she will think that I don't care.

Karen responded with:

But that is our own lack of comfort. It's hard to say 'I'm sorry, I don't understand you. Can you wait a moment?'

The group continued to think through the implications of their nursing practices for these families. They realised that they were always friendly, always nice, but they djdn't stay with these families long enough to care for them, there was always something else to do.

This project illustrated how the tyranny of niceness is being perpetuated. As Sophie said:

The women from non English speaking backgrounds are the ones that miss out. Think how many times that we stand in a room and talk to an English speaking parent [about what is happening to their child]...how many times, just in conversation [we discuss things with them]. We talk about different things [related to their health] all the time.

Anna interjected:

Yes and you pick up a lot of important information.

Andrea remarked:

You explain things at the bedside all the time to the parents.

Sophie commented:

Isn't it interesting that we don't value our own nursing work enough to think it is worth while to get an interpreter to do our bit [explain our work]. As soon as a doctor has got something to say we all say, 'Oh, we'll get an interpreter.' It is sad really.

Andrea continued:

With some people, by the time you get to the end of the admission interview, you have got a mate for life. You would not be able to do that with someone from a non English speaking background. You can't throw in the little bits in between that form a relationship or form a rapport.

As you can see, these women are beginning to think carefully about the specifics of their clinical practice. Working together they appreciated the value of having people from different ethnic backgrounds in the groups to challenge the taken for grantedness of their eurocentric nursing practice. Just when this group decided that they would use interpreters more frequently, Shan reminded them that they would have to make time for this. She also suggested that they needed to think carefully about how they could use the interpreters effectively as there were transcultural issues at stake. She commented on her own experiences as interpreter and as nurse:

I have worked as an interpreter of Japanese. I would find it the most frustrating thing because the person would always say too much. Then the person who I was interpreting for would say too much, too fast, and I couldn't remember it all. Some of the things they were saying were quite important and I just wanted them to slow down and say a little bit at a time. So sometimes, especially with the Japanese language, you have to change things around so that it does not sound rude because Australian [sic] and Japanese are very different types of languages in that Japanese is very polite. To change words around takes time and if it is a really difficult concept then you have got to think about it.

The comments helped the group consider how communication issues affected discharge teaching and how this probably explained why some children from families of non English speaking background were more likely to be readmitted to hospital. As Anna commented:

When you think of discharge teaching of an English speaking family, really we prepare them for discharge, or they prepare themselves for discharge, right from the word go, 'What is that medicine you're giving?' 'Oh, this is Lasix which makes them wee'. 'How long are they going to be on that?' and all that sort of thing, and by the time they get home they will be able to say, 'Oh, yes that is the Lasix and that is given twice a day. I remember that one.' But with the [families from] non English speaking background, they have not had that learning process over the last five or six days.

Over the past three years, these nurses have been restructuring their nursing practice in ways that make it responsive to the needs of children and their families regardless of their socio-economic situation, their culture, or religious background. This form of cultural change takes a long time. It is early days, and some of those days are very frustrating, but we are all starting to see changes in how we care about the health care roles, practices and structures in which we care for ill people and their families. It is a journey of discovery on which we have embarked in order to understand more about nursing. We are interested in understanding those superb instances of individual caring that regularly occur within nurse-child-family relationships, and how by thinking about the clinical rituals, practices, discourse, power relationships and reflective thinking, we can support each other to move beyond the tyranny of niceness to genuine caring.

3. Workloads, power and privacy

The taming of time

I am behind today.
Behind what?
Behind where I think I should be in my work.
Does it matter?
Probably not—I don't know what I am talking about really—we always
say that...we're behind or ahead.

Clinical nurses have learnt that they need to complete many
physical, technical and psycho-social activities in a day's shift, and
that they will not only have to do their own work but that they will
be expected to facilitate and co-ordinate the work of others. This
sense of not being in control of their own work load unless they
keep 'ahead' is a consequence of not having enough status in a
work environment and of participating in caring roles which make
constant demands—both occupational aspects of female-con-
structed social roles. Ideas of time are constructed in ways which
are evident in language—'ahead', 'behind', 'going well today', 'not
keeping up', 'off the pace'—and influence how nurses practice. As
one nurse reported:

I find it hard to sit still and let Mr J slowly chew each mouthful, especially
when some of it comes back out like a baby. I want to hurry him up all
the time, to shove it down his throat because I keep thinking that I am
wasting time. It's crazy when you come to think of it because that's
what I am paid to do. To see he gets enough nourishment and doesn't
choke.

The cult of efficiency can mean the end of quality time.
Deinstitutionalisation has been introduced with impressive
rationales but insufficient funding to cope with the large numbers
of ill people released into community care. This overburdens

community nurses so that no one ever has enough time. When an unexpected emergency occurs, community nurses can find themselves stretched to the limit chasing resources and providing appropriate care. One nurse, whose client load had increased dramatically both numerically and in the severity of the cases with deinstitutionalisation, commented:

I spent most of the day with this woman yesterday and missed out on seeing about seven people, which I have to do today on top of the others I was going to see.

Nurses based in the community depend upon excellent working relationships with members of other health disciplines. However when community psychiatric nurses require the services of a doctor to assess someone they often have to wait for hours. As one nurse suggested:

It took ages to get someone to come and see him and then the GP [doctor] was late, and the third [person] the psychiatrist was late and then I was trying to get a bed that wasn't available. They eventually got one in the forensic unit. I just can't believe how long it all takes. I'm sure if a doctor had to sit with that person for 4-5 hours it would get done in half an hour.

The suggestion here is that not only is the co-ordinating role time consuming for nurses but that time is an issue for medical practitioners who finish their clinic before rushing into the community to see a stranger who is acutely unwell. However the nurse is also suggesting that, if the doctor was expected to sit with an unwell person waiting for the appearance of the nurse, there would be changes made to the system.

Time is also an issue for nurses when they are attempting to provide consistency of care. One PAR group found that the consistency of discharge information provided to parents was related to the amount of time available to nurses to provide that teaching. An account from one of the group member's journal highlights this issue.

Coming back to a busy afternoon shift after having had days off, I was assigned a child in a hip spicas who was to be discharged that afternoon. After having talked with the parents for a while I got the impression that they were not as ready for discharge as I would have liked them to be. The mother was asking a multitude of questions such as, 'What do I do if he keeps crying at night?' 'Does he have to sleep on the Bradford frame?' Questions poured out in a panicky fashion, the parents, not being adequately prepared, were having doubts about coping at home. I felt inadequate, wondering how I would possibly teach them all they had to know in the short space of time left prior to their discharge, taking into account the busy workload I was already faced with.'

In fact heavy work loads, and the difficulties that these appeared to create, led the group to question whether the discharge education held enough priority in the unit. At one meeting, a group member succinctly summarised this point.

Because of my workload, I often feel guilty about not having enough time to spend with parents, doing discharge teaching. I feel that discharge teaching is not considered a high priority on the ward. This is reflected in the workloads we are faced with.

When we discussed this issue it soon became evident that proper discharge education takes time. The group members said that they often experienced difficulty finding the time to conduct effective discharge education. Within the limited time available, they felt that caring for the more immediate needs of ill people frequently took priority. There were times when they faced many sick children, a number of whom may require constant care following surgery, and who would only be in hospital for a limited time due to decreased bed stay times. The group members saw the problem with workloads as the constant demand to meet people's immediate needs. Group members often had little chance to provide time for discharge teaching. The problem of priorities and workloads is real but they are also replete with unexamined myths, control myths which can be deconstructed in a collaborative process.

Power relationships and nursing

I think of myself as powerless—so junior and always doing what other people want—even the patients. But it is only when I nurse someone who has been a patient often...you know, who knows the rules, their rights. It is only then that I see how much power I wield over patients without knowing it—well acknowledging it. This happened yesterday and I realised that I sometimes tell people things—manage what I tell them and when [I tell it]...because I want them to fit into my routines. That's the power/knowledge stuff you were talking about isn't it?

A key area of interest for many nurses is a concern with the exercise of power. Historically we have always talked about power as if it was a commodity—something that someone had and someone else didn't. Foucault (1972, 1982) has led the way to re-examine notions of modern power and understand power not as a commodity but as a relationship—not what someone has but what is exercised in a particular context. This is not to suggest that our opportunities to exercise power are the same. They are definitely not. Neither an alcoholic nor someone with a psychiatric illness is able to exercise power nearly as often as the doctor or the lawyer or the psychiatrist or the nurse or the social worker. Society sanctions the exercise of some forms of power and minimises the exercise of others. However the important point that Foucault raises is that we generally ask the wrong questions about power. Instead of asking, 'Who has power and who doesn't?' we need to ask, 'How is power functioning in this instance, how is it being produced and how are the relationships being structured?'

These power relations can be discovered within the intricate webs of human social relationships where power is produced. The quest to map the exercise of power in clinical nursing practice requires a rejection of polar oppositions—the either/or. We must trace a winding path with many byways and intersections through multiple configurations of power.

It is not very useful to say that doctors 'have' the power and nurses are oppressed by it in the health care system, even though all nurses have felt powerless in the face of medical power. We continue to speak of the dominance of medical discourse since medicine can be seen to dominate and limit nursing so often, and in such seductive ways. However power is not exercised in a vacuum and medical discourses are constantly competing with a variety of subordinate discourses in complex clinical situations. The discourses of medicine are struggling with discourses of nurses, patients, hospital administrators, an increasingly informed public and government departments who hold the purse strings and the expanding, threatening discourse of the law. Clinical nurses experience these webs of power, and when given the opportunity to reflect on and unravel the complexities, they easily identify the links between power and knowledge.

The exercise of power combined with knowledge in nursing is primarily analysed through reflection on language, meaning and cultural practices. So if we think of the differential exercise of power by both dominant and subordinate groups, for example medicine and nursing, we should also think of the forms of resistance evident in language and action. As one nurse reported:

The doctor told this mother she could take B [her son] home right away, with no prior warning and so of course she wanted to, and didn't want to wait around. And yet he [the child] was supposed to have medication, and we had to send to the pharmacy for that, and he was ordered a nebuliser, and we had no time to explain to her how to use it, and this little boy was very lively and hard to manage with the pumps. In here we had found out ways to manage that, which we wanted to show her, and when I told her we would need to explain it she said, 'Dr A said we can go and he should know'. So I went to Dr A and told him that unless he wanted to see this little boy back in hospital very soon he needed to go and tell the mother that she had to wait and couldn't leave until she had spoken with the pharmacist and the nurse. He was not impressed, but I held my ground, because this is something we had been talking about in the PAR group, and so, instead of just whingeing about him [Dr A], I decided to challenge him. We set it all up with the mother and she was really pleased in the end, and I was glad that I had seen that I could use some power for B.

As Foucault suggested, 'maybe the target nowadays is not to discover what we are, but to refuse what we are' (Foucault 1982:216). Feminist analyses are concerned with deconstructing the ways that women have been positioned in society and then reconstructing them by refusing the positioning and the roles which have been socially constructed. Nursing practice is shot through with gendered power relations. As nurses become aware of the complexities of the power relations in which they are enmeshed, they can also inform feminists (Maaresh 1986), who have largely ignored nursing as an arena of interest, about the micro politics of gendered power relations in nursing and health care (Oakley 1986).

Power and representations

Media portrayals of nurses as 'old dragons' or 'promiscuous, sexy young women'—mermaids and sirens—continue to recreate myths. These representations contribute much to the confusion of the nursing role. 'How can nursing be adequately represented?' is a question that requires considerable attention and one that can not be easily answered. Nurses are not a homogenous group and yet they have been shaped through their knowledge, skills, rituals and shared experiences to take on a healing role among the health care disciplines. The nursing literature strives to decide whether nursing is an 'art' or a 'science' and whether medicine 'cures' and nursing 'cares' in an effort to describe what it is that nursing is and nurses do (Dunlop 1986). And nurses are still not sure. There are too many answers and they are all right in part.

The print and electronic media still portray nurses in caps even though nurses have not worn them for years. Uniforms will continue to symbolise a nurse even though nursing uniforms are disappearing from many institutions. These signs are potent and typify the nurse in a way that is not apparent for most other professional groups who need to be portrayed in relation to the tools of their work for occupational recognition. Nurses need only to be depicted wearing a uniform. This carries the message that nurses, like the armed forces and the police, are people under discipline, who can be relied on in a crisis to carry out orders without fuss. However nurses have not been remunerated for this role in the way that other male dominated uniformed services have. As nurses begin to understand the way in which power is exercised through varying forms of representation and inequitable remuneration, they began to see how their own practices have been shaped. Nurses who become aware for themselves of the restrictions of expectations, stereotyping and institutional forms of representation can then explore what these things mean for the person who becomes a 'patient': they can understand the effect on a modest person of being undressed and washed by strangers; the difficulty for each Vietnamese person who is regarded as a clone of the others; the frustration for a sick person who is asked to repeat their health history again and again as they get represented in the different forms of documentation of various health professionals; the irritation of experiencing constant stereotyping, which is sexist, racist or ageist—or all three. An exploration of the competing subject positions of the nurse can help them provide care which acknowledges the various ever changing subject positions of others. The power of representations are embedded in habitual practices but can surface during the participatory research processes despite the very pragmatic focus of much of this research.

Power in the professional 'gaze'

However power is not only exercised through forms of re-presentations but also through systems of differentiation which codify the person into discrete medical categories. These become the focus of the professional 'gaze'—what it is possible to see within the restrictions of particular situations. A telling example of this was an experience of my own.

Recently I required a succession of eye operations. As the procedure was experimental the protocol dictated that only one eye is operated on at a time. After the second surgery on my left eye, I found that it healed well and looked fine but that the untreated right eye was deteriorating and looked red and swollen. I went to an outpatient clinic and experienced two forms of specialist gaze. The orthoptist took one look at my eyes, assumed that the red right eye was the product of recent surgery and went to put drops in it. I deterred her, she checked the chart and we agreed that my left eye needed the particular drops. The surgeon came in and looked only at my left eye as he knew from my chart which eye he had operated on. He was very pleased with its progress and asked if I had any questions. I asked him what to do with my red right eye. It was as if he had seen for the first time since he entered the room that I had two eyes on my face separated by my nose. He is an excellent surgeon with such a highly specialised gaze that he didn't even see eyes in the way other eye professionals see eyes. He saw only the eye which was under surgical treatment at the time.

The 'gaze' of the nurse encompasses many discreet and different things about the person, their condition and immediate environment. This gaze is much wider than the gaze of the surgeon, being much less specialised and much more integrated. However, the gaze of the nurse is also conditioned at times by what it is possible for the nurse to see. The nurse's gaze will sweep a room and notice specific details such as a buzzer that has fallen out of reach of a person. When visiting in the community the nurse's gaze will recognise minute changes in the condition of the person, or their living environment. However the nurse may miss what the relative sees about their loved one. In one participatory research group the nurses became aware that they saw people with asthma within a framework of expert knowledge and experience. This framework included the generalised picture of an asthma sufferer overlaid with a conglomerate of all the people who the nurse has experienced, and do not fit the typical picture. It gave the nurse a possible picture of the next person with asthma they encountered but also a set of expectations which sometimes led the nurse astray. One was that the relative would not understand the asthma picture as well as the experienced nurse. They discovered that this may mean that the nurse discounts the relative as a source of informed knowledge of the particular pattern of the person's asthma pattern. The parents of a very young or disabled child will generally interpret signs and symptoms differently from the nurse and will become an expert in the reading their child as they have a very clear and narrow focus. Acknowledging and validating the parent's gaze in relation to their own child became a focus for the group.

Who owns the space?

An interesting phenomenon in current hospital philosophies and mission statements is the claim of providing care not just for the person in the bed but also that person's 'nearest and dearest'— sometimes labelled 'family centred' care. As babies and children are generally part of families, the Royal Children's Hospital in Melbourne, Australia, has participated in this trend and has rhetoric in its mission statements which support family centred care. A recent policy decision enabling a parent to sleep in the bed next to the child patient, when the unit is not full, is a demonstration of the hospital's concern. Health professionals talk about the bed and its surrounds as being 'a home away from home for children and their families'. The unit staff encourage families to bring familiar things from home to decorate the hospital bed space and make it appear more homely and less threatening to a small, bewildered child. The space around the bed is notionally allocated to the child and their family for the duration of their stay; however the actions of staff often demonstrate something very different. It is apparent that nurses and other staff pay lip service to the idea.

When observing, we noticed again that nurses enter rooms and walk diagonally across to the beds as if the space was one large room and they had right of egress to any part. In contrast, visitors move down the centre of the room and enter the space around the bed of the person they are visiting as if there were invisible walls.

There was an interesting spatial question at work here which related to the familiar way that the nurses used the space in which their work was located—taking control of all the space without regard for any notion of the person's space.

The rhetoric of family centred care was also not reflected in the architectural design of the unit spaces. The mismatch was obvious with families who opt to stay all day and/or overnight. They are often in the way of nursing activities or seen as disturbing other children and families in the unit. In other words, it is not possible to change just the rhetoric of mission statements and to announce a hospital unit as a family centred area without thinking very differently about space. Moreover, when nurses have been involved in designing new areas in health settings, these areas still carry the same contradictory messages about how the space is to be used.

Changes may be made in the placement and height of cupboards, desks and beds, but essentially the result in western cultures is easily discerned as a hospital ward. This occurs because the taken for granted assumptions remain tacit so the eurocentric, medically dominated, individualistic culture of health care is replicated with different colors and new furnishings. But how could this be otherwise unless these contradictions are sought out and explained?

It was as a novice ethnographer charting the world of hospital practices I first noticed how the same space was used differently by people with different status and occupation and began to understand the meanings for nurses and for those in their care—be they patient, family or friend—at the micro level (Street 1992a). Later work challenged me to also regard the implications at a macro level for the hospital administrators and funding bodies.

At the micro level, ritualised behavior occurs which is a curious mix of the habits of normal social intercourse with regard to privacy and the traditions of open surveillance which are part of the hospital. Watching visitors enter the symbolic space around a hospital bed is to see them avert their eyes from anybody else as soon as they have identified that they are not the person they are seeking. Then there is the tentative pause at the end of the bed waiting for recognition and some form of encouragement to come nearer, if that is possible given the circumstances of the person. Then the entry to the space is made in a manner that suggests that the person in the bed has some control over the space around them. The advent of visitors usually is marked at this point by spatial rearrangements of what is essentially a cramped space—even in a private room—to accommodate the visitors and provide more resemblance to a living room than a bedroom. This flurry of welcoming activity, with minute adjustments to the environment, mirrors the normal activity which surrounds the welcome of unexpected guests in a family home.

These private rituals contrast with nursing routines. Nurses spend a great deal of their time one to one, but they also spend time on general surveillance—the nursing 'gaze' at work. When nurses walk into the unit with the intention of checking on the patients, they usually stride into the centre of the unit and either just observe each person, checking on a multitude of things apparent only to the skilled nurse, or speak loudly to someone from the centre of the room, 'How are you feeling now Mrs Jones?' 'Mr Smith have you had a shower yet?' When the focus of their work is on a task or interaction with a particular person then nurses invariably walk diagonally across the room to the person's bed as if the bed was just another piece of furniture in a large room.

The contrast between the actions of the visitors and the nurses is instructive. The visitors act as if the large room was in fact a number of small private rooms with invisible walls, whereas the nurses act as if they were in a large living room with people in beds rather than chairs. This has significant implications for the person in the bed and for their friends and family.

It is important to understand the spatial arrangements of nursing work and the effect that these arrangements have on nurses. As I have argued elsewhere (Street 1992a), nurses' work is done in public view. In her book *Gendered Spaces*, Daphne Spain argues that it is common for occupations which are essentially designated as women's work to be conducted in public:

> Women's jobs can be classified as 'open floor', but men's jobs are more likely to be 'closed door'. That is, women work in a more public environment with less control of their space than men. She contends that the female constructed and dominated occupations of secretarial work, teaching and nursing are conducted in public spaces whereas male dominated and high prestige occupations conducted in the same areas occur in private offices and clinics. Doctors have the opportunity to conduct their work behind closed doors, nurses don't. This lack of spatial control both reflects and contributes to women's lower occupational status by limiting opportunities for the transfer of knowledge from men to women (Spain 1992:206).

Although many health professionals in hospitals do their work under the public gaze, it is apparent that the higher status the occupation the more privacy is afforded behind closed doors. Hospital cleaners, porters, trades people, aides and nurses carry out their work almost exclusively in public spaces under the public gaze. Other occupations work somewhat in the public gaze but also have their consulting rooms and meeting rooms and private offices and secretaries to protect them. These 'open-floor' occupations are characterised by little control of space, resulting in a lack of privacy, lack of control over knowledge, and constant surveillance. Women typically engage in work that is highly visible—to colleagues, clients, and supervisors—and subject to repeated interruptions. The spatial conditions under which women work both reflect and reinforce their lower status relative to men's work (Spain 1992:227).

These specific characterisations of 'open floor' occupations are evident in nursing. They not only have implications for nurses but are paralleled in the experience of people who are ill. The parallels are informative as the spatial behavior and experience of nurses can be contrasted with the experiences of patients.

In my previous work (Street 1992a) I found that this need to constantly deal with intimate situations in public spaces meant that nurses became either visible or invisible to others depending on the person, the place, the time and the forms of symbolic representation—the uniform or the stethoscope. This differential visibility also affected how nurses used space. Once they become accustomed to working under public scrutiny and learning what to see and what to ignore they can learn to behave in ways that would be unacceptable in other social contexts. The relative of a patient told me:

In a sense what happens is that people sweep into a room as if it is public property, and they talk about you and your family and all sorts of things as if you are public property. There is not the sense of we are entering almost what is someone's home for the moment. Many of the women try to set up some of those things, try to make a space that feels a little like home for their loved one, and nursing and medical staff invade it and do not show any respect towards this person and their space.

In a participatory research group during a discussion on this topic one nurse said:

We were taught to respect the patient's space, et cetera, when we were in college but on the ward...Well no. Who would ever conceptualise the patient's personal space? It's not something that I've ever heard anybody talk about on the ward...referring to someone's personal space.

And another continued:

Yesterday when I was doing some 'obs' two nurses came into the room, and one yelled out for someone. A physio came in and started talking at the top of her voice, and when the nurses came in, they immediately took over the space as their own.

Paradoxically nursing work is also invisible work despite being carried out in public places. Much of the skill and art of expert nursing is invisible to the uneducated eye of the lay person and often to the educated eye of the medical staff. Many expert nursing decisions are made through informed but invisible observation. For example, final year nursing students recounted how they had been taken into a psychiatric unit and watched as the nurse sat at a table and read the paper while the people who were unwell, were engaged in a number of meaningless and bizarre activities. The zealous students challenged the nurse during the debriefing session which followed demanding to know why she just sat and read the paper instead of working. Her response was, 'What would you have me do shut up in this room for hours—stare at them all the time?' She then went on to give a detailed account of all the activities in which the participants of the room had been engaging and explain her understanding of the reasons for them. The chastened students learnt a valuable lesson about the invisibility of skilled nursing observation.

Nursing work requires the kind of skilled surveillance in which the ill people are very visible to the nurses. The nurse is held responsible for the well being of these people throughout the shift and this responsibility is passed on to another nurse at the end of the shift. Each hospitalised person is extremely visible in terms of documentation in the medical file, in the filling up of a hospital bed, as someone who is discussed at handover or on the medical round, as someone who needs to be fed, washed, medicated and treated. However this kind of visibility carries the contradiction that many patients claim that nurses miss seeing things that are important for their welfare. Family members often stay in hospital because they feel that their loved one is not visible enough as a whole person to the myriad health professionals who briefly engage with parts of them. The person in effect becomes invisible to nurses and other health professional if they are not responsible for them at that time and in that space. As one father said:

My son is not as ill as the others in his room and doesn't set off alarms all the time so I wonder if the nurses and doctors really see him. I wonder if they remember he is there half the time. He is still a frightened, sick boy.

Being both visible and invisible depending on the situation and the personnel involved can limit the way nurses think and the way they nurse. It will also limit the possibilities for 'seeing' the experience of people who find themselves both very visible in medical terms but invisible in other human terms.

In the same way as visibility and invisibility are spatial matters for nurses and for ill people. Lack of privacy is another spatial issue encountered by both nurses and patients. Units generally do not provide private space for nursing staff to conduct research, education and administration. The assumption is that these activities can either be carried out at the nursing station under public scrutiny or away from the unit. As nurses are also generally required to be on the unit during their shift, they are not provided with the same spatial incentives to pursue research and continuing education as medical staff who are not confined in the same way. This lack of private space for nurses to study and write near their patients and colleagues is a strong disincentive.

The lack of privacy impacts on people in two ways. Patients do not have the benefit of nursing care which is informed and enhanced through continuing nursing education and research, nor are their own privacy needs as well understood and acknowledged. The religious requirements of a Middle Eastern culture can pose difficulties for a culture where hospital space is available only for medical technology. A Muslim who wanted privacy to conduct his daily prayers in hospital was sympathetically understood by a group of nurses whose research had been haunted by a similar quest to find a private space where they could discuss confidential data.

The effects of space on the way nurses think and act becomes part of the taken for granted world of nurses' experience of hospitals. It constitutes a series of acceptances and expectations about patients and their privacy rights. Nurses who have been carefully trained to cover body parts with towels to ensure modesty when they give ill people a full wash may not offer the person the same privacy when discussing medical and lifestyle requirements, or making racist, ageist, or homophobic statements in a loud voice in front of others. The living room becomes part of the working environment where nurses exercise the power to structure it according to their own values, needs and desires. Spaces become dark as nurses pull down blinds for 'the afternoon nap' in spite of the wishes or needs of patients and visitors. Spaces become noisy because staff call out across them, or rip off paper towelling at wash basins near sleeping patients, drag furniture around, or forget to turn down monitor alarms.

Surveillance and lack of privacy are not the only spatial matters which affect nurses and patients. The third characteristic of gendered space is the potential for women's 'open floor' work to be continually interrupted. Nurses learn to arrange their work with repeated interruptions although this is rarely acknowledged. Experienced nurses speak about passing on this aspect of nursing culture to novices as part of the process of helping them to learn to be organised, to manage to get their work done in the shift. Nurses talk about the stresses of never having enough time. The advice novices receive is sometimes about prioritising their nursing activities; more often it is about ways to get the work done as quickly as possible in case there is an emergency. Real unexpected emergencies are few and far between, but interruptions are a constant and often unacknowledged reality.

The culture that is being passed on is a culture of coping with the unexpected, and that is mostly constituted through interruptions. Clinical nurses know that one thing they can count on is that they will be continually interrupted. Another thing not so easily perceived is that they in turn continually interrupt others and interrupt their own work if no one else does. This emerged in a research discussion group from a nurse who was engaged in participant observation:

In that instance the people who came in walked right through things that were going on—commented and interrupted. Made some loud comments and interrupted. One of them talked across everybody else, when they could have come around and spoken to the nurse. The other nurse came in and interrupted what was happening for the child, which disturbed the child, and then went through, past the parent, and through again, and spoke to the nurse who was undoing the stitches, which meant the whole thing had to sort of slow down and stop, and apart from the kid screaming and all that sort of thing, there was this other thing going on which could have been dealt with two minutes later when all this was finished.

I have often walked into a unit to talk with a nurse and, seeing that she was busy with a patient, I have waited outside the room. Other staff come past and chat with me and then ask, 'Who are you looking for today?' and then tell me to go into the room. I will tell them that I can see that the nurse is busy and that I am prepared to wait so that I don't interrupt her work, but this is rarely accepted. The other staff constantly want me to interrupt and tell me, 'It's OK, she won't mind, go on in'. When I explain again that I will wait they will often go in and interrupt the nurse and tell her I am waiting. The nurse will also find it strange that I haven't interrupted her.

When this problem of interruptions is suggested to nurses they immediately agree and some will talk about how they are interrupted and the consequences for their work. Of interest is not the notion that nursing work is constantly interrupted by others, but that if others do not interrupt nurses, then they will interrupt themselves. Being interrupted is so constituted and inscribed on the bodies of nurses that they learn to move rapidly from one thing to another and find it difficult to sit at one task in one place for a period of time without interrupting themselves by thinking of other things to do. This is evident with nurses who engage in post graduate education and affects how nurses participate in research.

Nurses become so used to being interrupted at work that they also interrupt each other's work all the time. Nurses who have been sensitised to this through clinical participatory research are amazed at how many trivial interruptions occur in situations such as when a curtain is round a bed during a procedure. Questions like 'Who's in here?', 'What's going on in here?', 'Are you going to first tea?', 'Have you got the keys?', are just a few of the common ones identified by the nurses.

This rite of repeated interruptions influences how nurses act with and toward patients and their visitors. The living room attitude is demonstrated when a nurse feels able to move into a room and interrupt a conversation between a sick person and a visitor to ask a question that either can wait or is unnecessary. Nurses interrupt patients who are dozing to ask them questions which do not require an immediate answer but which 'I just wanted to get done now while I think of it'. If the person was doing the same thing in their own bedroom at home the nurse would think twice about interrupting for such trivial reasons. But working in the spaces constituted through nursing culture creates different public and professional ways of being for nurses.

This discussion of the effect of space on nurses and their patients has so far been conducted at the micro level of local knowledge and actions. However these stories are also forged at a macro level which demonstrates the localised political effects of party political decision making. To illustrate this interrelationship I want to recount a story and give it repeated readings.

A unit manager came into my office to discuss some research possibilities for her unit. She had recently returned to her position at the hospital after pursuing further studies at university. We talked about how her course had alerted her to the inconsistencies between her newly acquired nursing philosophies and the habitual practice which re-emerged when she found herself back in the unit working with others who expected her to continue in the old ways.

At the unit meeting held on the previous day, she had talked to the staff about changes in work practices and how everyone now needed to think of themselves as family centred nurses and not just as neonatal nurses focused on babies and their needs. The discussion continued about how families were to be welcomed on the unit and particular attention was to be given to helping mothers who wanted to express breast milk for their babies. On the day after the meeting as she made her rounds she became aware that one nurse was caring for three very ill neonates in a space designed to hold three isolets and equipment. However in that small area were the families including toddlers who were running underfoot. At the end of the shift the unit manager commented to the nurse that she must be tired as it would have been difficult dealing with all those families. Upon reflection the unit manager saw this as an instance of her own inconsistency, where her comment to the nurse demonstrated the habitual unit attitude, which was at odds with the newly espoused unit philosophy of delivering family centred care. This unit manager blamed herself for giving conflicting messages to the staff.

At a micro level the unit manager may have been inconsistent as inconsistency is a normal part of change. However I gave her another reading which looked to the wider political implications. This was an accommodation and resource issue. The hospital had changed its philosophy from 'we care for kids' to one of care for ill children and their families in line with community expectations and government health policy. The changed philosophy had been incorporated into the corporate plan. However no changes had been made to the physical spaces where this care was to occur and no more personnel had been appointed to help nurses deal with the competing demands of sick children and their healthy brothers and sisters, particularly when toddlers are not in the siblings' creche. Neonates have never required much space to nurse as their isolets are small. Until recently the unit did not have any babies who were intubated, so there was no need to provide ample space for extra monitoring equipment, and the space needs of nurses have always been seen to be provided for at the nurses' station and a small meeting and tea room. Now the nurses were expected to care for more seriously ill babies in the same confined area and accommodate all the space requirements of the family at the same time. This meant organising their work with more demands, greater noise level and more confinement of their movements. Under these circumstances the unit manager's comment was entirely appropriate. It had been a hard day for the nurse, and by implication, if there had been no families present, it would have been much easier. This situation can be understood as a hospital resource issue whereby the staff are required by policies and protocols to practice in a way that is extremely difficult in the space allocated. However public hospitals are funded by public money through health departments, which have policies and funding formulas that do not match the space and resource needs. The same inconsistency experienced at the micro level of the individual nurses is also apparent when the policy and planning sections of the health department are charting new directions for health institutions at the same time as they are reducing funding in real terms. It would be simple to suggest that the health and community services departments are the culprits here. However they are part of the political system and are dependent on the policies and funding of the government of the day. So we could blame the government—a common enough but futile exercise—and this would still not answer the space needs of families with hospitalised children. The government has access to limited resources which are not always wisely spent, being generally spent on whatever community needs will provide the most political gain for the party in power. This is true of the state of Victoria but it is also true of other places.

The competing demands and machinations of the political system affect how one nurse feels at the end of the day when she goes home blaming herself for her inability to do the impossible. That she does so is because the issue of space is not understood as a cultural and gendered issue that impacts on our lives in unacknowledged ways—at a micro and a macro level.

4. Establishing a participatory action research group

Participatory research processes in nursing have been established and modified over the past six years during my work at the Royal Children's Hospital and through university teaching, community-based research and national and international consultancy.

PAR requires that nurses take part together in the process of doing the research. The rationale is threefold. Group members bring a variety of interests, knowledge, skills and experiences to bear on the issue under investigation. The group provides a context for critique, challenge and validation. As PAR is directed at cultural change and improving a given situation, a group of committed people have more chance of making informed choices and implementing them than an individual. This last point is particularly relevant because PAR is not hierarchically imposed. Rather, it is based on the assumption that the people who are affected by a given situation are best placed to determine how to change it and make the implementation process work.

Getting a group started

PAR groups may be formed in a number of ways and for a number of reasons. It is important to identify the reason for the group as PAR is challenging and time-consuming and requires energy and commitment. If members are being coerced into participation or provided with a topic of concern to others, the group will have difficulties in giving the time and effort required.

Composition of the PAR group

Only through the process of 'owning' the question and the intervention strategies can groups function effectively. It is important that group members deal with issues in their own practice as a clinical nurse, nurse educator, or nurse administrator, and not set up groups designed to change other people. Such establishment is important if group members are to work creatively with the issues as they emerge for themselves as individuals, for others in the group and for those people who are seen as their critical reference group. As nurses rarely work in isolation from other disciplines it is not uncommon to have other health professionals participating in the group with their nursing colleagues.

Another concern is the power relationships which are introduced through the composition of each particular group. In some groups nurses involve the unit manager, others prefer to keep the manager informed of their progress. Many unit managers are keen to support the process but realise that some of the clinical problems are better resolved by the people directly involved. Other unit managers have joined groups and have found that rosters mean that they are the only person who can attend regularly. That means they can exercise power over the direction of the research by virtue of regular access to knowledge concerning the project, reinforced by the institutional power they habitually exercise. As one perceptive unit manager wrote:

Equity is a difficult concept to realise in any group. Vested interests, power relations, structural constraints and territory are some of the many considerations which have to be thought through if a group is going to function effectively and give voice to all. As unit manager my position in the group was clearly not at the same level as the other registered nurses. Having a dominant voice and being in a relation of considerable power with the rest of the staff, my membership in the group had a significant effect on the way it functioned. The presence of another senior male staff member and his relationship with me set up a particularly powerful dynamic which on many occasions threatened to disrupt the group functioning. The very skilful manipulations of the principal researcher salvaged many meetings from total fragmentation.

It became obvious to us all that the research could not continue and issues would not be successfully worked through while I remained in the group. During my one absence from the group the other staff discussed how I was exercising power to run my own agendas. The researcher and I discussed this and I agreed to absent myself from group meetings on a regular basis. I would be updated on the progress from time to time through a report back from staff. This decision was seen to be entirely appropriate and the group functioning was restored, those voices which had been subordinated were given space to be heard.

Another issue in the establishment of groups is the issue of gender. Male researchers and male unit managers working with groups of female nurses need to address the forms of patriarchal power which they may be inadvertently exercising over the women. In the same way race may also be an issue where predominantly white Anglo-Australian voices in the group are privileged over nurses from other races, particularly Asian women.

The way that institutional nursing work is constructed around rostered shifts and regular movements of staff to other wards or other hospitals may mean that the group members have had no real contact with each other prior to the first meeting. This has implications in the way group members 'hear' and understand each other's stories and comments. It is beneficial if some of the taken for granted attitudes and assumptions which participants hold can be elucidated during this establishment phase. If unfamiliarity with each other appears to be a potential difficulty for group members I ask each person to give a thumbnail sketch of their own professional life, making links between their specific history and their current attitudes and experiences.

Such a potted history might be told around questions such as:

- What were my earliest associations with nursing?
- How did they shape my original conception of what it means to be a nurse?
- Who have been important influences on my nursing history and why?
- What are my hopes for this participatory research group?

As biographical sketches are forthcoming the group learns to value each others' individuality and the contribution each can make to the research enterprise. Discussions on these histories have been very helpful and illuminating for the individuals and for the group. During one discussion with a group who began their 'training' during the late 1960s I mentioned my own political activities in relation to protest against the Vietnam War. One nurse commented that during those days when people were taking to the streets in their thousands she was not even aware of Vietnam or the protests. She was busy making sure her cap was correctly folded and the stripes on the bedspreads were lying evenly and going in the direction specified by matron. Other nurses echoed this experience of being part of a total institution which cut them off from the concerns of the community by shift work, endless lists of tasks to learn and knowledge to acquire by rote.

After a discussion with members of a graduate class about this group's experience, one graduate student sought me out. She explained how this had been illuminating for her as she often felt that she had lost some history as she had no knowledge of key events in Australian political life, much to the amazement of her husband and his friends. She had traced the date of one such political event and discovered that she was in a new ward doing night duty and totally pre-occupied. Newspapers and news bulletins did not reach her consciousness while she was learning to cope with new routines, new drugs, new patients and the stresses of night duty. This nurse was glad to understand a phenomenon which had puzzled her and to know that many of her colleagues had experienced the same historical blackout during their training.

Stories such as these help nurses in new groups understand how the rituals and routines of their nursing training and practice have shaped their view of the world around them. Recent graduates bring different histories and expectations of nursing practice and the research process. It is important that these are explicated at the start of the group so that participants find some common ground and understand some of the platforms from which people may speak.

Establishing positive research attitudes

Although groups tend to get together because they share a common concern it is helpful to encourage the group members to keep their concerns in perspective. Nurses are no different from any other occupational group who find it easier to identify problems rather than achievements. It useful to ignore the question, 'What is wrong?' and replace it with the question 'What is it like when things go well?' This question is followed by, 'Why doesn't this happen all the time?'

This moves the emphasis from a negative, self-defeating focus to one that acknowledges creative nursing practice and accesses the cultural constraints of nursing such as role conflict, power relations, medical dominance, or time constraints. This positive perspective is important, as my experience with nurses in clinical and academic situations has convinced me of the goodwill of most nurses in regards to the interests of their patients or students, and of the effects of structured institutional repression and violence on the potential for acting on that goodwill. I would support the statement by East and Robinson (1994:61):

We found little evidence that nurses were resistant to change and much to suggest that many were anxious to improve standards of care. What was against them were structural factors with an economic basis; the tremendous day-to-day fluctuation that defied all attempts at continuity of care arising from financial constraint and crisis management.

The situation is mirrored in academic settings in Australia and New Zealand where I have found it rare for academics recruited for their clinical expertise in one area to remain and develop advanced knowledge in that area in the academy. Too often decisions on teaching specialties are made on the grounds of need resulting from economic limitations and nurse scholars become weary and negative about the chances of bringing about change.

It is important to provide a positive platform on which to ground understanding and change. I ask research participants to give recent accounts when their practice made a difference for someone else. These accounts are very important as they not only provide valuable research data but fuel the group's vision of what is possible. In this manner the participants and the critical friend/researcher are able to identify common experiences and attitudes, along with specific differences, which will shape the way problems are conceptualised in the project.

Forming a PAR group from a group of colleagues is the beginning but it does not turn clinical or academic nurses into researchers. The next step is to familiarise the group members with the process—preferably through a workshop which gives infor- mation about the strategies and processes along with the chance to begin to isolate a common concern.

Identifying an area of common concern

When research participants establish a group they identify common concerns and isolate a researchable nursing issue of interest to all the members. The nurses in one group formed because they were concerned about the fact that few mothers established breastfeeding with their low birth weight babies. As one staff member commented:

The culture of the ward in which we work prevents breastfeeding happening a lot. Just today at 11:30 a.m. the ward clerk found me and said, 'Can you come out here quickly?' I went out and here is this mother, who I'd never laid eyes on before, who was distressed...tears pouring down her face, sitting at the desk. I thought, 'Oh no, what's the baby's name, what's it here for and what am I going to do?' Anyway

I said, 'Would you like to come down here and have a talk?' So we went down the end and I said, 'What's the matter?' So she just let it start pouring out...

So after listening to her story I went down to the room and said to the nurse, 'What's happened?' and she answered, 'She's just run out'. So the staff were in a panic, but, of course, nobody went out to find out what had gone on. She had come in and the nurse said she went to explain what was going on, but the mother had just panicked and run outside. So they were left there thinking, 'Oh god, what have we done' and I said, 'I think we should take the baby out, disconnect it from the monitor and take it down. Give the mum the baby to cuddle and see if she wants to breastfeed'. Everyone said, 'No you can't do that the [medical] round's coming in here now. We have told the mother she has to stay outside because the round was coming in here.' It's because, on these days, the rounds come around and everything stops for the rounds. That's the way we are, we're there, and we have to have the baby ready for the doctors when they come around, and that's the job that we have to do. I would have been exactly the same in that nurse's position. But because as the person in charge I was removed—I was outside of the situation—I could say, 'That's not the issue. The issue here now is that this baby goes out to its mother and spends time with its mother, that's the most important thing. They [the medical staff] can come and do the round and do this baby last.'

I'm guilty of it myself. I have done it, and if I was there by the baby today, I felt that I would have done the same thing. It's just those little things we had to re-think about.

Concerns such as these need to be shared if effective action is to be taken to improve the situation. In this instance I was approached by a small group of nurses and requested to help them start a breastfeeding action research group. They recognised that the culture of the unit did not support mothers of very low birth weight babies to establish and maintain breastfeeding. Stories such as this relate to specific contexts but share common themes with the stories of nurses from very different contexts. Many nurses experience the effects of medical dominance on their practice in such a way as to limit their actions. Nurses who work in high tech contexts under obligation to administration for 'patient throughput' report pressure to focus on the technical needs of their patient to the detriment of aspects such as nutrition, comfort, patient education or social relationships.

I have found that the key themes underpinning many clinical nursing stories are very similar, although the context and the specific dimensions of the issue are unique. One group concerned about effective discharge education from the orthopaedic unit began in this way:

The CRAG (Clinical Research Action Group) came into being as a result of concerns I had relating to the number of telephone inquiries received from parents wanting information or reassurance following their child's discharge from the orthopaedic unit. As an associate charge nurse on the unit, I was often the person who answered the phone and had to deal with these type of telephone queries from parents who had difficulty caring for their child at home. These phone calls made me feel both angry and guilty concerning what I believed was a lack of adequate information being provided by nursing staff for parents prior to their child's discharge. An account from my journal highlights the issue and my feelings in relation to one such telephone call from a parent: 'Today I received a phone call from a very distressed mother of a child who was discharged two days previously in a hip spica, after a fractured femur. She seemed angry and frustrated and was appealing to me for help. "She has been screaming with pain and not sleeping for the past two nights. I've tried panadol and panadeine, but it doesn't help. What can I do?" I suggested that if the child was still in pain then perhaps she should bring her back, but at the same time reassured her that these concerns were quite legitimate. I felt in many ways helpless to know what to say to this woman. At the same time I was angry that I had received the brunt of her anger, which somehow implied that we had failed. Also the frustrations of receiving numerous calls of this type made me feel very guilty about the lack of information given to parents prior to discharge'. This and other similar queries prompted me to call a staff meeting to discuss my concerns related to discharge education on the ward, and find out if these concerns were shared by any of my colleagues. From that meeting it was evident that there were a small core of nurses who had also experienced problems in the area of discharge education and planning, and who were interested in working to improve the effectiveness of our nursing practice in this area. Out of this meeting the CRAG group was then formed, and we decided to meet on a regular basis using the PAR methodology to address the issues which had been raised [An unpublished report of the CRAG group].

A group of nurses from another unit joined a project examining aspects caring for families from non English speaking backgrounds because this was a concern for them too.

In our ward we have quite a lot of people of non English speaking back ground that come in...We're a ward that gets emergency cases that only stay for a day or up to three days, and then they go home...and we've actually found just on a ward basis, that the way we treat non English speaking background families, really wasn't up to scratch at all. Then when something actually came up onto the ward in regards to La Trobe University doing some research into our use of interpreters and how we treat non English speaking background people on the ward...there were a few of us that actually pricked our ears, and thought maybe, five of us should get involved in that project.

In this instance an area of concern was identified in some preliminary research conducted by the ethnic health unit and an earlier NESB PAR project conducted in conjunction with the school of nursing at La Trobe University. When further funding was procured, staff employed in units which had not been involved in the earlier PAR project were given the opportunity to see if they also wanted to be involved. After explaining how the ward became interested in volunteering to join the funded project, the nurse went on to discuss her own motivation to join the group:

I wasn't actually doing anything [at the time]. I did a paediatric course the year before, so I felt as if I wasn't really doing much study, or really getting involved in a big way within the hospital. So I put my name down, and then it was just a matter going to a meeting with J, and finding out what she was actually intending to do with the research project. I was quite interested in what she had to offer, so I joined up. But I think it was really a need thing for me. I hadn't really got involved in any research as such during that year, and our ward really needed some development in that area also.

This form of development, where a concern is identified and either wards or individuals are invited to join, is common. However it is also possible that a group of nurses may know about the benefits of PAR and decide that there they would like to use it to understand and improve their situation. The initial storytelling process often reveals a number of interests. Then the participants can decide which is worth investigating in their research.

The reconnaissance

When an area of concern has been established and a group of nurses formed to investigate it, using the PAR process, a reconnaissance is conducted. What is a reconnaissance and what has it got to do with research? As one group commented:

It sounds like something from the army, you know, like someone going on a reconnaissance mission to check out the territory before the army moves on.

A reconnaissance is an initial fact finding process which involves a systematic exploration of a specific situation in order to provide an informed basis for the development of the first action plan. It may also provide baseline data for later evaluation of the effects of the research. In the reconnaissance stage we encourage individuals to meet to describe their concerns and interests, exploring with other group members their ideas and experiences and the possibilities of the situation. Out of these discussions members can then collaborate to identify a thematic concern, that is, a substantive area which is of concern to all and upon which the group members intend to focus their strategies for change.

Evidence of the current situation

In most research projects when the topic is clear the next step is to investigate the literature. Since PAR is directed at deconstructing and reconstructing the habitual practices inherent in a situation, there is a need to develop a clear picture of the situation as currently understood and experienced. The literature will not address the specific needs of a group of nurses or academics in a particular setting so it is useful to leave a literature search until after some initial descriptive data has been obtained.

I have found it useful to ask participants to describe the current situation carefully and collect information from their own and other people's experiences.

Participant's accounts

Writing down stories of each participant's experience as regards the general concern enables other group members to understand the nature and extent of the issue in their own context. One nurse who was in a group concerned with developing more effective doctor-nurse working relationships, recounted this situation:

I returned from the tea break to find a toddler in my care was missing from the cubicle. I asked everyone where he was. No one knew the whereabouts of the child. I paged the doctor and the parents but neither responded. No tests had been scheduled so I checked all over the ward, and then the cafeteria, in case the parents had come to visit and taken him there without telling anyone. I was getting frantic and I had five other children to care for in that section. Finally the doctor answered his pager and admitted that he had scheduled a chest X-ray and sent the child off with his parents without notifying anyone on the ward of his departure or destination.

When the nurse told this story her colleagues immediately told similar stories and the group was then able to focus what had been a very broad topic down to a more specific one, which related to the problems of how doctors' orders are passed on. By teasing out this situation, the nurses were able to design appropriate action plans to address their specific problem.

Participant's accounts of colleagues' experiences

Accounts of situations told to participants by others who share their concern from within their context or from a different context may illustrate the same issue. Any change is difficult to implement and more difficult to maintain. If a group of nurses want to improve a situation in their work context, it is valuable if their colleagues also recognise the same issue. Many nurses have also found it useful to their understanding of an issue to find out about the experiences of colleagues dealing with the same thing in other contexts. Often in a PAR group nurses will recount stories from their friends, flatmates or relatives who are nurses elsewhere. The story of medical staff not notifying unscheduled tests was confirmed by others. That nurse also told a colleague's story:

The EEG department rang to ask why a child had not arrived for their EEG at 1015 hours. The nurse caring for the child was not aware that an EEG was booked as there was no information concerning an EEG booking provided in the patient history or nursing notes, or given in handover. The EEG department requested that a nurse be present during EEG as they did not have sufficient staff to stay with the child. The child's parents were not visiting at the time, thus the nurse had to stay with the child for over an hour in the EEG department. This nurse had a workload of five other children also. The doctor requesting the EEG had not notified any nursing staff concerning this booking, thus the nurse was not organisationally prepared to leave her workload of five other children for over an hour, at a moment's notice, at a normally busy time of the morning.

This account validated the concern and demonstrated the effect, not only on the nurse but also on her colleagues who had to cover for her work in the ward and the children, who received less concentrated care during that time.

Experience elsewhere

Accounts of previous experience from other places such as units, hospitals, universities or communities where the situation is managed differently may be useful. Nurses often underestimate their own experience as a resource. As most nurses have worked in many different places they often have encountered the same issue in different ways. These experiences provide both insights and specific information. In one project a nurse who had worked in another country was able to access some information from that country to help the study. The material proved invaluable as it stopped a group of nurses spending a great deal of time developing a protocol which was in use in another place and could be readily adapted.

Formal reports

Information can be collected from formal reporting procedures through the institution or community management committee, from conference speakers, from meeting resolutions or policy directives. The discrepancies between theory and practice are evident in the rhetoric of formal reporting processes such as organisational mission statements, policy documents or the minutes of meetings. Nurses often neglect to examine these documents and therefore lose the opportunity to use them to strengthen their argument. An examination of unit communication books, of nursing notes and other less formal communication modes are revealing for not only what is recorded but the manner of recording and also particularly in relation to what is omitted. Nurses have found that their issue has been raised repeatedly in the unit's reports but that no one has acted upon it. Likewise nurses have found that nothing has been documented on a regular nursing issue although it is talked about repeatedly in the staff room. Academic staff report spending a great deal of time talking about the how to teach their material creatively but that the subject files contain outlines and reference lists which reflect only content and not process. The real issues of nurse education are invisible in the documentation.

The historical background

It is important to set the scene. Nursing issues do not appear out of nowhere; nor are they created by specific individuals. Issues are contextually grounded in the history and culture of nursing as well as being situation specific. The historical development of the issue will demonstrate both its relationship to the wider nursing culture and community while also highlighting the specific local situation.

The literature review

The literature review includes an overview of the current research on the topic. It provides the participants with the opportunity to find out what others have investigated and written about in relation to the chosen topic. Keeping abreast of current literature is part of professional practice. Although reading the literature has been encouraged at an academic and senior management level, rarely are institutional or practical supports provided at the clinical level to give nurses the time and the skills to do this. The researcher may need to initiate nurses into the mysteries of the library and provide them with the confidence and skills needed to conduct computer literature searches and some critical strategies with which to analyse articles.

Developing research consumership skills

The skills of identifying appropriate key words, conducting computer searches and using research literacy to select what articles are valuable is part of research consumership skills. These skills are necessary if nurses are to be able to assess adequately what they find in the literature.

One novice group reported back to their colleagues on the literature in a written report to the ward meeting:

We went to the hospital library in search of articles on how other nurses dealt with the issue of developing an effective handover. Many of the articles we read were expressing much the same concerns and problems which were discussed at our action research meetings. Common concerns between hospitals in America, England and ourselves involved ineffective handovers due to no specific format and the giving of irrelevant information about patients.

The group went on to identify very specific information which was relevant to the concerns of their topic:

Boredom and lack of interest from the afternoon staff was noticeable when lengthy handovers occurred. Another contribution to this situation was especially heightened when handover was conducted so each morning staff person came and spoke to the others at handover—a situation we had found on our ward—and much time was wasted by staff sitting waiting for other staff to come to the room. Repeating lengthy information about long term patients to regular staff members was also an issue. Although the articles expressed concern about similar problems which we encountered, there was no article which related specifically to our problems or the changes we want to make. It was interesting though to compare the different techniques and changes made by different hospital wards relating to their handover and how to utilise time effectively.

The group then wrote about key articles of interest and listed the strategies which had been adopted in other situations for consideration in the discussion at the research meeting.

To turn this level of work into a research literature review takes further work. A literature review is a sustained evaluative argument and so the material needs to be organised from general to specific points in a way which presents a case for the conduct of the research. Novice researchers can become confused between a literature review which synthesises the content from a variety of articles and an annotated bibliography which presents a sequential discussion of each article reviewed.

The nursing research reported in the literature is often produced through quantitative research with the researcher framing the question in a specific way which enables the researcher to measure or predict something. The concern of quantitative research is to generate findings which can then inform the work of nurses in a variety of contexts. These findings may illuminate some areas of a PAR group's concern but may not be structured in such a manner as to help address the specific contextual question which has been generated though a desire to improve current practices. More often the issue which has been raised by the nurses from their own practice has had very little attention from nursing researchers. This is because the concern as it is articulated is based in the practical problems which nurses deal with in their daily work rather than the study of medical or other phenomena which interest nursing researchers generally.

The cyclical nature of PAR means that the focus has the potential to change a few times during the life of the project so a sophisticated literature review may not be possible or necessary for a PAR project. Instead a number of brief literature searches on different aspects of the topic may become necessary to get basic information as the project develops. Then a larger literature review may be developed to support the reporting stage of the project. I find it helpful to think of a literature review as a funnel shape where the broad overview of the main interests and methods of the literature concerning the topic are presented. Then those articles which raise more particular concerns or illustrate key concepts are presented. Finally the research which is most closely allied to the question and methods proposed are discussed, synthesised and evaluated. It is helpful to structure a basic literature review around various questions discussed below:

- What have other nurses and health professionals written that relates to this concern?

Nurses sometimes respond with the answer, 'Nothing!' when confronted with this question. This may be true about the specific details of their topic, particularly when the question relates to a new area of investigation. One student could not find any articles which directly related to her interest in how nurses dealt with the ethical issues of nursing donors and recipients of organ transplants. She needed help to expand her selection process to include other literature relating to the ethics of organ donation but also the lay literature which related to the experiences of families from the perspective of both donor and recipient.

Conversely, because nurses have not been careful enough in the selection of key words a literature search may produce far too many possible entries. A group of nurses interested in the management of orthopaedic pain found more than nine hundred articles in their first search.

- Is the research in the literature helpful to our problem? If so how?

It is important that nurses assess the value of the literature to their specific problem and not to include material which is interesting and related but does not shed light on the problem. It is also important that nurses identify whether an item is a research article or an account of someone's good ideas. Many articles published in nursing journals are the result of student projects and so it is important to discover if the writer(s) simply investigated a topic and came up with some recommendations or if they actually put the recommendations into action and evaluated them. Research literacy skills are valuable to enable nurses to ask critical questions of the articles they encounter to see if the research design is plausible and appropriate. Furthermore, a familiarity with the different levels of journals and the kind of work they include helps nurses decide if the material is helpful. Union and other journals directed at a wide readership solicit articles which are short, of universal interest and make easy reading. Serious international research journals will solicit peer reviewed complex material of narrower interest range written in a more sophisticated style. Both are useful resources for nursing projects but their value needs to be understood in the context of the needs of the research.

- Where are the gaps in the literature in relation to this problem?

When we are clear about what has been written about our topic then we can identify the gaps. These gaps may be methodological— that is, the topic may have been investigated in a way which does not meet specific needs. It is not very helpful to know that large numbers of people do not comply in the regular use of their drugs for hypertension if the clinical problem relates to how to deal with the re-admittance of people who are non-compliant to treatment regimes.

- Why is our problem important for us and for other clinical nurses/health professionals?

It is vital to establish that the problem is a valid concern as it is difficult to expect anyone to participate in research of little worth.

The first action plan

When the reconnaissance is completed and some exploration of the relevant literature has been undertaken, the group members are ready to plan their first action.

The action plan itself is a simple whom, when, where and how statement of the specific action. However the development of an appropriate action plan requires the kind of careful and critical attention that is given to the development of an hypothesis or question in other research methods. The action plan can be developed within a structured framework with a series of questions.

The rationale

An advantageous way to articulate the rationale is to answer the simple question, 'Why do we want to change the situation?' It is important that each group member is clear about why they are undertaking the proposed action. A lack of clarity can undermine motivation if there are challenges to the action by others. When answering this question it is also important to consider whose interests are being served by the continuation of the present situation. In many cases nurses discover that the action is being taken in the best interests of medical staff or administration rather then those for whom the nursing care is provided or for the nurses themselves.

The specifics of the plan

The action plan can be clarified further through the question, 'What do we want to change?' Answering this question involves breaking down the particular group's strategies for change into single actions. There are often so many issues for change thrown up by the reconnaissance that group members have difficulty deciding where to start and which issues should have priority. This situation can lead to conflict within the group as members vie with each other over what they do first. In order to deal with this situation, group members may elect to divide up the activities among the different group members. Although this may be seen as a way of getting things achieved quickly, dividing up the activities like this may also work to fragment the group and reduce the power of collaborative action. It is also poor research practice. If a number of activities are mounted at the same time, the results achieved cannot be evaluated separately and so no assessments can be made about their effectiveness. It becomes impossible to argue forever that particular actions were effective or ineffective because they cannot be isolated from the effects of the other actions mounted at the same time. If what we do is to be recognised as sound research practice, the action plans need to be made, monitored and evaluated systematically. If this does not happen, the group is not engaged in PAR but in participatory action of the kind that happens haphazardly whenever a few people get together and decide to change something. The reason we argue for PAR is that the cyclic dimension means that, rather than giving up—which is what usually happens when good ideas are implemented but later discarded—the process enables group members to understand what happened and how they can move forward, modifying their plans as they learn more.

The feasibility of the plan

Establishing PAR within an existing clinical, educative or administrative role requires some re-organisation of the structuring and priorities of that role. In order to examine the feasibility and effects of the proposed action we ask the group members to consider the question, 'What constraints am I facing?'

This question is essential if the intended action is to be instigated successfully. Many enthusiastic novice researchers err on the side of thinking and saying, 'Oh she'll be right', letting enthusiasm generate an implicit faith in their capacity to make things happen. Without a sober assessment of the constraints there can be no informed decisions concerning which are negotiable and which will restrict the group. The main limitations are usually:

- time to conduct the action plan
- space for interviews, focus groups, etc. and data storage
- communication within the group and with key staff
- resource support.

When these and other constraints have been identified, we ask the next questions. 'Which of these constraints are negotiable?' It is worthwhile spending time understanding the possibilities and limits of the constraints which have been identified. This then leads to the question, 'How will we negotiate around these constraints?' leading to a further decision concerning who is the most suitable person to negotiate.

The question, 'Who will be affected by my actions?' alerts us to the fact that actions produce changes for more people than just the performers. The ripple effect became apparent to a group of nurses planning to help mothers of critically ill babies establish breast-feeding. The nurses recognised that time spent providing education and support to the mother would be spent away from other clinical responsibilities. This would impact on the load carried by other staff members, and if this was not negotiated with them, it might cause dissent and could damage the possibilities of collegial support for an action plan, which all the staff agreed was appropriate but had difficulty implementing. Since nurses felt anxious about the effect on their colleagues of undertaking this additional teaching role, their action could also impact on the parents who might sense that they were 'a nuisance' to staff. As a result the parents might become unnecessarily concerned about the care their child received.

As nurses identify the potential positive and negative effects of their research on those around them they can minimise problems such as the one described above.

In order to assist nurses to be realistic about the possible consequences of their action both unintended as well as expected we ask them to consider, 'What could go wrong and how can we deal with that?'

This is a vital question and yet it is one that participatory researchers often ignore. When this question is posed group members often say, 'Nothing', and show surprise that we want to pursue this further. As social contexts are notoriously unreliable in terms of constant predictable responses it is important that the nurses recognise how and why their actions may be thwarted. Enthusiasm and optimism are not enough and can lead to disappointment and frustration rather than understanding and critique.

Data collection strategies

The final question about the development of an action plan focuses on the relationship between action and the monitoring process to collect evidence of the effects of the action, 'How can we systematically collect information that will enable us to examine the effects of this action?'

The choice of data collection strategies depends on the specific research questions and the most effective ways to answer them in research terms. For example, in a study investigating the knowledge and decision making processes of mothers in relation to the management of their children's asthma we chose to combine quantitative and qualitative research methods. Unlike some researchers, we did not choose to combine the two methods because we believe that qualitative research methods are 'soft' research and require 'hard' quantitative research to validate or support the findings. Rather, we were seeking to obtain different kinds of knowledge and so chose the methods designed to best provide us with answers to our research questions. We used an interviewer administered questionnaire to survey a representative sample of our target population to collect demographic data, establish asthma severity indices and delineate the knowledge that the sample population held about signs, symptoms, triggers and drug compliance. This enabled us to involve a large group and to make some comparisons and generalisations from the findings. The method enabled us to determine what knowledge people had, and the resources they obtained it from; it didn't tell us what processes were effective in their learning. The quantitative study told us what steps people had taken in their decision making, but it couldn't tell us how they made the decisions and how they were influenced in their decision making. For these questions we needed to use indepth open ended interviews and qualitative analytical methods.

We could use quantitative methods to discover how many parents discontinued the use of steroid preparations but it was through the qualitative methods that we were able to find out, for example, that one mother discontinued these drugs because she mistakenly believed them to be anabolic steroids. She knew anabolic steroids were illegally used in sport and believed them to be dangerous to her son's health. When this mother's worry was discovered we found that other parents shared her anxiety, a concern not considered before by health care staff in their asthma education programs. In this way we can see that different forms of inquiry match different questions and generate different answers about a particular issue.

Writing about data collection and analysis for PAR creates its own hazards. Traditionally these activities are described in textbooks in neat categories with cautions about objectivity and rigor or subjectivity and validation. Such accounts comfort those seeking recipes for the right way to do things. However they can be very discouraging to those enmeshed in situations that are subjective and dynamic and do not lend themselves to traditional notions of objectivity and rigor. As Poland (1990) suggested about her own action research project, it is often very difficult to stand back and see what this kind of research looks like when you are engaged in it.

Decisions about the appropriate form of data collection depend on whether it is important to be able to say how many people have had a particular experience or whether the meaning of the experience is important regardless of numbers. Usually a variety of data collection methods is used within any project.

The need for reciprocity in the research designs means that it is common for data collection to be interactive—and interactive designs are not easily described because they involve action and relationship. Interactive methods are particularly important for nurses in clinical, educational and administrative practice. These people choose to become involved in research on top of their full-time work because they have problems they want answers for. They usually do not have the luxury of thoroughly exploring the dimensions of a question or a hypothesis without responding to the needs exposed by the investigation. I have found that nurses could not explore pain management without becoming aware of things that could be done to improve its management. Consequently, they didn't take kindly to research designs which expected them to keep collecting data and ignore the implications of the information they were accumulating. It was because we knew that the nurses would take action regardless because of their concern for their patients, that we formalised the process. The action was clearly elaborated and defensible, implemented and monitored systematically, and subject to careful scrutiny and analysis.

Taking action

When the group has decided on the appropriate data collection strategies it is ready to embark on strategic action. The action needs to be designed to continue long enough for the group members to be sure that the effects that they are observing represent the typical picture. This means that the time span for the action needs to be decided with enough flexibility for it to finish early or continue if appropriate.

5. Building a research culture

First I want to make a detour to address three areas—funding, management resources and structures, and ethical consent—which form the basis of the concerns raised in workshops. These areas are important precisely because they are not given much attention in accounts of projects. However my experience in establishing participatory research projects with nurses carrying heavy clinical loads has taught me that the conditions for developing a research culture depend on the establishment of some basic prerequisites.

FUNDING AND ITS IMPLICATIONS

Who pays for participatory research projects? How can you get funding when you have to compete with quantitative projects which easily fulfil the research and ethical criteria of institutions where no one has heard of PAR? These questions are commonly asked by nurse administrators interested in establishing participatory research but aware of the need to identify and fund the costs involved. In contrast with other research methods participatory research can be regarded as relatively inexpensive. This is evident in its successful use in community development by self-help groups and community activists. It does not need big budgets for experimental drugs, expensive equipment, chemicals or other laboratory requirements. When participatory research projects are conducted by practitioners on issues that concern them about their own roles, relationships, language, work practices and structures, they may not need access to sophisticated technical support for data collection and analysis. Nurses in these kinds of projects may use tape recorders and computers to record and transcribe the rich oral culture of nurses in stories and debates at group meetings, but such equipment is not essential.

However there are always costs in any research. Consumables such as stationery, computer disks, tapes and photocopying costs

must be charged to someone's budget and it cannot be assumed
that the unit or community health center can absorb all the expenses
in its clinical budget. According to one unit manager:

If you were putting up a budget to do a project in your area and you
wanted the grant to have three research fellows to do this over six
months, you would also need to put in your budget the transcription
or typing costs or secretarial support to this amount [sic] as nurses
are not employed to be typists.

Another unit manager agreed:

There were a few people that wanted to do some research around
the ward with the orientation program, and they wanted to review it,
and they wanted to get it typed up. One staff member spent a whole
lot of time trying to learn the computers on the ward, and she wasted
hours, really hours, and then finally I told them about D on the fourth
floor, who was a secretary, so they went down and found her, and
the work she did after that was amazing. Because they had found
someone to do the typing they weren't getting frustrated any more. It
made a difference to the work that they churned out for about three
months after they found D…D was absolutely tearing her hair out
with the work that was going down there, but the stuff that was coming
up to the ward, was amazing.

This unit manager also recognised that with adequate research
support the nursing staff could enjoy achieving something within a
reasonable time frame.

And it all just highlights to me that because research is so new to
nursing, if the nurses have a pleasant experience with it, it's also the
best possible thing they could ever do. And you know…give them a
good experience, and they'll keep doing it.

Many projects generate phone/fax expenses, transport expenses,
library costs, conference fees and costs for binding reports. Nurses
generally underestimate such expenses as do experienced researchers. Unfortunately few funding bodies are prepared to cover
actual costs, expecting the institution to be able to finance some of
the hidden administrative costs. Some funding agencies will allow
the addition of a percentage of overheads to cover leave entitlements,
medical insurance or other add on salary costs, however other
funding bodies, such as the Health Research Council of New
Zealand, expect that this will be covered by the institution.

The greatest research cost is personnel. Despite some evidence
from self help and third world contexts, my experience with

participatory research in academic, clinical and community settings in developed countries suggests that this form of research generally requires a skilled critical friend and researcher. This is certainly the case if a group with no research background is going to learn to use the research process and the skills involved in it. The critical friend is not only a guide, but provides the 'outsider' view that appears essential if the work is to lead to genuine cultural critique and theory building. As one nurse research participant explained:

But you certainly need to have key people around the wards I think as a referral person. People that nurses can go up to and say, 'Look, I'm thinking about this, but I don't know how to get it started' or 'I've started this, but I'm stuck, I don't know where to go next' or 'Do you know how to?' Many people probably don't know how to do a literature search in the library. They probably don't realise the amount of literature and stuff that's around, 'cause they just don't know how to access it.

In this instance the nurse is identifying the need for the researcher to be both an outsider to the specific role of the nurse but an insider to the work context. As an outsider the critical friend or researcher can provide research skills development, project direction and cultural critique. As an insider they can appreciate the contextual limits and possibilities of the situation.

This need of a critical friend to provide information has led me to apply for and receive funding for projects to appoint researchers to work with the nurses either in an institutional or community setting. Academic feminist nurses who are interested in collaborative and participatory research with clinical colleagues can find that the negotiation processes take time and effort which is not rapidly rewarded in the form of publications. Most nurse scholars also find that the strong emphasis on teaching and the demands of clinical teaching make the need imperative for resource support in terms of typing and transcribing or research data collection and analysis. Research administrators may be useful for a clinical project when the participants have learnt some research skills but don't have the time or the computer skills to prepare material for analysis or dissemination at all stages of the project. Administrative support is also very useful in community settings where nurses may operate in isolation from each other most of the time and carry a heavy case load.

A further funding matter should be considered when participatory research includes people who are financially vulnerable. This is the necessity to apply for funding to pay people not only to conduct interviews but maybe to pay people to be interviewed; to refund any transport expenses for people on low incomes; or to pay costs when participants undertake activities in their own homes.

MANAGEMENT FACTORS

Although less easily identified, priorities and lack of administrative support, time, space and resources are as much funding issues as visible equipment, consumables and personnel. Participatory research groups established by community nurses, academics and administrators will encounter similar problems. However these groups usually have more autonomy in structuring their work and more control over their diaries and priorities than nurses in hospitals who have the added complications of shift work and a large changing population of colleagues to research with.

Setting priorities: the need for management support

Participatory research in any busy academic, community or clinical context needs effective support from management. This does not just mean lip service but constantly giving high priority to research activities as is done for clinical, teaching or administrative activities. And this support needs to be put into action and not just announced at meetings or in performance appraisals. This support is essential and it does not matter whether the administrator is actually interested in research or not:

From a management point of view I support it and the staff got all the support they needed. I'm not a great one to read research or get involved in it. However I do support it and the staff can do as much as they like. That's fine.

Sometimes a manager gives lip service but no flexibility in relation to time out of a busy schedule. Staff cannot accomplish their research goals in time and may lose funding or enthusiasm or both. As one clinical nurse commented:

When M was in charge she'd try on that day to get someone extra to work to cover us and stuff. That wasn't always possible because we didn't have the full support of the charge nurse, and without that, it just makes it impossible, really.

In academic contexts constant lip service is given to the need to research and publish but it is rare for this to be written into academic workloads in a way that means that time is actually allocated to it. This attitude has its roots in the fact that most university nursing departments have evolved from colleges and polytechnics where teaching was the main emphasis. As a result there are many fine nursing teachers but few fine nursing researchers—although there are many nurse scholars of considerable ability who could do excellent work if their time was prioritised differently. The constant changes in policy and funding priorities instigated by government departments has meant that hospitals, community settings and universities have increased the processes of bureaucratic accountability without re-allocating staff time.

Implementation of findings

Research projects take time. PAR projects are particularly time consuming because they entail cycles of action and evaluation which involve the negotiation and participation of the key players. When a PAR project is planned it is essential that management and other staff, or clients who may be affected by the implementation, understand that the process will take time to complete. It enables the researchers to fine tune the action plan through a cycle of implementation and reflection followed by problem reformulation and further implementation and evaluation or reflection. This means not only time to do the preliminary investigation but time to trial a number of action strategies until the issue has been resolved. A unit manager who has had a few PAR projects on her unit commented on this aspect:

With projects it's very important that there is an end result seen, otherwise the nurses look back and think, 'What we've done has been a waste of time.' So I believe from a management point of view, if I'm going to support, or participate, or allow them to participate in a research project, I have to be prepared to allow them to implement the change throughout. There's no point in them coming up and saying, 'This is what we've found S', and I say, 'Well, I'm sorry we can't do anything about it'. That, to me, would be absolutely devastating to anyone who has spent a year researching it. So, you've got to be prepared...even if you may not agree with it...you've got to be prepared to allow them to make their mistakes, allow them to implement it, and work through the problems that might arise. Different things happen...there's lots of little things changing throughout the whole year. So, I think it works better if they actually see the end result rather than the whole thing wasted.

Administrators also need to recognise that they may not like to deal with changes to the habitual practices on their units as many of these practices suit them. However as it is the clinical nurses who will be implementing the changes to their care, it is important that administrators acknowledge that there is more than one way to achieve good nursing care and that their ways may no longer be appropriate. As one administrator acknowledged:

Some of the changes I haven't agreed with, but then I don't have to make it work. And all year they've worked through it and come up with another system that suits them, and they think it is better for the patients. And I may have to admit that it is.

Administrative support of this kind is essential if clinical nurses are going to make an impact and develop a clinical nursing research culture.

Prioritising yourself

The constant modification of the institutional and community structures within which nursing is taught and practised means that it is not easy to develop a research culture. The conservative environment of the hospital is a challenge for any participatory research as is apparent from these comments:

Nursing research sort of started about three years ago, I think, and when it first started people were quite anxious about it, and there was a lot of animosity towards nurses who were involved in research by other nurses because they saw the research as not being important. They saw it as just a waste of time, and they saw it really as something that wasn't productive or useful.

The attitude of peers often produces unwarranted feelings of shame or guilt. When research is devalued in any setting, it can lead the researcher to feel defensive. I still struggle with my feelings about being absent from my desk even when the university supports my research and I have encouragement from senior staff. Meetings, teaching and general administration make more immediate demands on my time and I have to convince myself to do what I urge others to do—prioritise my research activities. My feelings have been echoed by nurses in many forums. One clinical nurse described her feelings like this:

As nurses part of our culture is to feel guilty. So we used to feel guilty about the time that we were spending away from our patient or how we had to rush in the morning so we could go to this research meeting. But in time we decided that we really had nothing at all to feel guilty about and we'd feel more guilty if we weren't attending these meetings, trying to change things.

Feeling ashamed is not the only concern. There is also a need for nurses to see that engaging in nursing research is part of their professional career path whether they are clinicians or academics. This is important motivation to persevere with research activities that are monotonous or seem unrewarding. As one nurse who wants a future as a clinical researcher suggested:

Obviously the interest varies for me as well, but, creating a kind of research structure and career path lends itself to fostering research, on a more concrete kind of level.

Allocating research time

Nurses need to be creative and realistic in apportioning time for research inside a busy schedule. In hospital, meetings and meal breaks interrupt every shift. The interruptions mean nurses are reluctant to have further breaks particularly when they are nursing people during a short stay. The demand for throughput means nurses have little enough time for discharge education in addition to routine care.

Rostering, shift work and research

What constrains us is our rostering...and things like that make it very difficult to conduct research and to, you know, try and get our groups together.

Participatory research processes require staff to work collaboratively. Time is necessary to meet regularly to report back on the contributions of individuals to the project and to work as colleagues on the research. Staff often have to be inventive and committed to get the time together. One nurse spoke of her group's commitment to communication concerning the research:

We would always make sure, whether it was at a tea break or if we could get some formal time out from the ward, we always made sure we got together once a week, just to talk about something, an issue that had been raised, or something on a personal level that was worrying us, and that was always documented when we had these meetings and what the meetings were about.

Things such as unit amalgamation during holiday periods, shifts and regular staff vacations create disincentives to maintaining the momentum of research as in this account:

We were committed to meetings basically, two to three weekly, depending on how we felt we were going, and that was fine. We did have an hour there where we could leave the ward and sit down and discuss it in quite a free manner and not feel as if we were needed back on the ward. Then our ward and another actually amalgamated over Christmas-New Year period, and so that meant we basically found that our meeting, and the whole research project, really virtually stopped, because we were quite busy. So really not much happened over consolidation, which was about six weeks.

Momentum is often difficult to re-establish particularly with the further complication of leave, as the story continues:

Then we've gone back to the ward, and we've found it very difficult, because one of the nurses has been on night duty, one of the other nurses has just gone to Africa, yesterday, so it's been hard to get together; and also because of the shift changes we're finding that we're going to split lunches, which we weren't before. So, we found it more difficult to actually get away from the ward, just because of the timing of things in the ward.

In clinical settings, research time needs to be structured into rostering procedures that will provide both individuals and groups of nurses the essential time to meet and engage in research activities. In academic settings the same stream of interruptions occurs but for classes, clinical teaching and meetings. Academic and clinical staff speak of being overwhelmed by the sheer volume of commitments to be finished before work could begin on research and the effect on the quality of work produced. Some women report that the burdens of family responsibilities, on top of a heavy teaching load, makes research impossible. An academic colleague commented:

Most of the nurses teaching here are women and the majority of them have families to deal with. For many of us we deal with the triple burden of marriage break up, demanding children and needy, frail, elderly parents. We know how to teach nursing so we get through the day shift, but then we face the night shift of family responsibilities and higher degree studies, and then this push to do research and to publish. Many of us have never done research except for qualifications. I know we have to do it and we would like to have the time to learn but we just feel swamped. There are just too many calls on our lives.

The pace is mirrored in the clinical area. One nurse described a typical experience like this:

It was at times very difficult to get time off the ward, and that was hard because you'd have to run around in the mornings and get everything done just so you could go to lunch early, or not even have lunch, and then, you know, come down and try and sit at these research meetings and get your thoughts clear, and you'd be thinking, 'I've still got six lots of nursing notes to write, I hope someone's doing it, I hope they haven't forgotten'. They've gone to afternoon tea, there's no one to take over my section. All that sort of stuff would run through your head so you weren't very relaxed about going to the research meetings.

However not all the research work can be conducted in time snatched during the shift or the academic day or during the nurse's own time. Systematic research work requires sustained attention as well. It is only possible when the staff members are given time to focus on research activities. Academics and clinicians alike need to be able to spend whole uninterrupted days on their research and at times, whole weeks. As a senior lecturer told me:

You feel pretty helpless really, with the lack of time you've got to do it. You have to do research—it is part of our bread and butter as academics and yet I find when I finally put aside a research day I have to deal first with my electronic mail and the messages on my answering machine and the mail in my box and then respond to the colleagues and students, and it goes on, and I get to the end of the day and think of all I didn't do. I need to be able to have an uninterrupted week to do anything reasonable.

It is unreasonable to ask busy nurses or busy scholars to add research to their existing workloads. The imposition of research that way needs to be resisted until another way forward can be negotiated. It must enable the redistribution of tasks to add some free time for research.

Integrating research and management

Administrative support for research is not only evidenced in priorities and time allocation, but can been seen when there is an integrated approach to the conduct of research. In the clinical area or in a community health setting, an integrated approach is a valuable way for research to become central to the work of nurses. Research projects require managing and therefore it is possible for individuals in a unit to collaborate on research projects from a number of perspectives. Two people could legitimately hold different management responsibilities in relation to the one project but from distinct viewpoints. One person could be accountable for the research design and another for procuring the funding and managing the resources. This may present some difficulties in terms of collaboration but could advance the clinical unit in terms of its overall function. It also recognises that different skills are required for success.

In academic settings administrators need to identify specific skills and interests in their academic staff and support their further development. This is the case for excellent teachers, for staff with administrative skills, for researchers and for writers. Combining the skills of staff into research and teaching teams can enable expertise and excellence to be developed in a number of areas.

Managing research resources

Nursing research is something we have to do and it gives more credibility to nursing.

The introduction of the nursing research needs to occur within a structure which:

- Identifies priorities
- Assesses the institutional resources and procures adequate budgetary support
- Develops competent and ethical protocols
- Identifies specific skills necessary and the means to develop or procure skills
- Identifies research performance indicators to evaluate research productivity.

Performance appraisal is necessary to hold administrators and their staff accountable for the nursing research in their area.

Accommodation requirements

Suitable accommodation for research is essential. Although most participatory nursing research activities do not require laboratory space or much office space there is a need for a place to hold confidential meetings, read and write, conduct interviews, and store files and equipment. It is often difficult for clinical and community nurses to be allocated space as research is not seen as integral to their role. As one nurse commented:

When I was doing the breast feeding study, we used to conduct our meetings in the treatment room, and of course, every time you know, every Tom, Dick and Harry would walk in, and you couldn't conduct a meeting, and as a result of that, we then started to move our meetings away from the clinical setting, so it's still in the ward, but it's down, right down the other end, away from interruptions, and it's in a closed room.

Clinical units need to provide a suitably furnished home for research activities which enables staff to meet and to work without interruptions. Accessible storage space for documentation and reference books is essential as is a lockable cabinet for confidential records and equipment such as tape recorders, computer software, etc. Many nurses who work in the community occupy limited, shared office space and have even greater difficulty than clinical nurses in acquiring suitable research space. Academics may have access to a research center which provides specialist research resources but may not readily be able to find a place for participatory research meetings in either the university or a clinical site. Dedicated space is valuable as it provides the opportunity to develop research skills in an environment which supports a culture of investigation.

Developing research skills

The only way to get nurses to do research is to teach them the skills. They all have to value their work enough too to want to research it.

Learning research skills is not only a matter of time to attend skills workshops. Nurses need the opportunity of informal and formal courses. However, in many instances, informal and formal research training is neither valued nor recognised in the clinical arena. Unlike medicine, where the career path expects and rewards clinical research along with clinical practice, clinical nurses often have to leave the clinical area for academia if they want to pursue research. Yet PAR is for people to use to investigate and improve their own situation.

But you see, for the medical people, they get time off, resource support, and when they get their MDs or something, they can go in and get jobs. They've got the capability to ask a lot more money, to apply for bigger funds, to have a lot more options in terms of career and all those sorts of things which aren't in the clinical nursing area. The options are to go and do your degree, your higher degrees, to go into teaching other nurses, but not to stay in the clinical area.

In order to consolidate clinical nursing research activities, unit staff who have basic research skills and have demonstrated a commitment to research on the unit should be given the opportunity to apply for scholarships.

I mean, T's got a first class honors degree. And was being pushed to go on and do a PhD. And she decided she needed to get some more clinical experience. But, you know, you don't want to just ignore someone like that, and give them no recognition. That is what she felt happened. She went away, got her first class honors degree, paid for it all herself, and nobody said 'Boo', so there was in a sense no recognition that this person had put a huge amount of work in to actually improving herself, and she's still, you know, Grade two, Year two, sort of thing…I actually…That's why I thought, the doctors have research fellows, why can't the nurses.

good idea

Nursing research scholarships could function to provide selected nurses from the unit with a paid day of research activity each week. The clinical nursing research scholarship holders could engage in some of the following activities:

- engage in a unit based research project towards a graduate qualification
- provide a research assistant role for the project(s) on the unit
- develop a proposal for funding
- write up the unit research for publication
- write a literature review for the unit research project.

A nurse who had been employed one day a week to support the researcher on a funded project that had a number of PAR groups, commented on her experience in relation to the need for research scholarships:

I think that would be fantastic! I find coming over here with R one day a week great. At least you spend the whole day focused on research, you're not spending an hour, running out from your section, all flustered, and then you've got to sit down and get your head together and try to think about the project and then run back, knowing that you've got to run back to the ward again and finish your notes, or do whatever you have to do before you can go home. So I think that a scholarship to allow a person to have a full day to just spend on their research would be a very viable option. I think you need that time to sort of, you know, be a researcher for a day, get out of the clinical setting, because I just don't think you can focus properly otherwise. And we were allowed to have days out when we did our PAR study, and they were our most productive days. We'd sit down, we'd work out what we'd done, and we'd be able to write up our reports and do things like that. Yeah, it was much more efficient. I think that would be a great idea...Plus, hopefully, these people can, hopefully get a publication out in their own names, which will help them with their CV, and will help them if they want to do further study.

Nursing research scholarships could be used to reward staff who have made a significant contribution to research at the hospital by enabling them to travel to do further research, to present papers at national and international conferences or to do some specific research study program.

F and H started off with their action research project, and they've written an abstract to present at the International Paediatric Conference. I was surprised. When the abstract for the conference came out I just said something like 'Why don't you write it up?', and they were just so keen, I thought they'd say, 'Oh, no, we've done enough', you know, but they were quite keen. I actually got their abstract there on time.

This comment is encouraging because it demonstrates that when some nurses who have been supported in research activities are given the opportunity to present their research in an international forum they will respond enthusiastically.

Unit communication

Communication of research needs and activities has been identified as a major problem. Nurses often speak about the difficulties they have in letting other staff on the unit know what is happening with their action plans particularly when not everyone is involved in nursing research or passionate about it.

We always came up with lots of issues that needed to be addressed and none of them were simple. They always involved other people.

Communication was not only a problem with other staff.

One of the hardest things that I found was communicating between ourselves and actually having that time to sit down and say, 'look, this is what we're doing'.

Heavy work loads, clinical teaching and shift work also affect the communication strategies which are necessary to disseminate research information, particularly if action plans are to be implemented. This problem is often underestimated by novice

researchers who make assumptions about their capacity to connect
with their peers, as is clear from this account:

Julie wanted to know how does she get all the other staff together to
tell them where they [Julie's research group] are at with their project.
She's going to have a meeting. So I said, 'We only have seven people
on today, how are you going to get the other fourteen that we've got
employed?'. It's a real problem disseminating information and also
decision making.

Another problem in communication occurs in any context where
the membership changes from meeting to meeting. Different people
make different decisions. This situation is a problem for the smooth
functioning of hospitals, community programs and universities. One
academic elaborated the difficulty he had getting his research
participants to agree on a suitable action plan:

I've found...because you have a group there, and they all want a
particular thing, so they make a particular decision, and the next group
come along and it will be a different lot of staff, and they say 'We
don't want that'. And you'd have different people fronting and they're
changing the plans all the time. It is so frustrating.

Communication is a constant issue for participatory research
because of its component of collegiality and collaborative endeavour. It needs to be addressed constantly to make sure that the
decision making processes remain with the group and are not
usurped by individuals who have better access to the information
or who happen to be in the right place at the right time.

I have found that it is essential to recruit a research group who
will be committed to the project, to schedule all meetings well in
advance and to predetermine all communication strategies. Some
groups find that if they tape record the group meeting then any
member who missed can listen to the tape. This means that the
absent member not only reads the outcomes of decision making
processes in the research notes but hears how the participants used
the information they had to make the decisions. This has been the
most effective intra-research strategy. This kind of regular
dissemination of research updates needs careful attention and
administrative support.

Another effective but very time consuming strategy to improve
the communication on clinical units, and in the wider community
of interest, has been regular research newsletters. These provide
detailed progress reports of individual research projects with

participants, topic, rationales, accounts of current findings, implementation plans and future directions. In order to ensure that these are read by staff, the compilers must make them interesting and accessible while covering enough material to educate staff on the current and future work of the research team.

Establishing forums where researchers can report back the progress to staff can also be an effective form of communication, but forums are often difficult to organise with shift work or teaching timetables. Nurses have to think creatively about ways to overcome the difficulties. Some nurses organise a succession of meetings over a few days to attempt to cover most of their colleagues. The meetings may be formal seminars as in universities or informal meetings conducted by a group of nurses on a unit. One nurse described her experience of setting up informal forums and communication strategies:

Well actually, it's just been ward meeting, and we did it with night staff as well as day staff, and it was just an informal forum asking them what they thought. Throwing some questions to them and saying, 'This is the kind of thing that we're wanting,' and getting feedback from people saying, 'Yes, well we do', or, 'No, we don't', or, 'Gee, I didn't know you could do that', that kind of thing. Other than that, having a resource folder on the ward, available to everybody, to know that they can go to look at it and be free to look at it.

This nurse found that her strategy of informal forums for different shifts and keeping a resource folder of the current research information worked effectively on her unit. But when the group decided that they needed to investigate how other wards were dealing with the situation, she found it much more difficult:

I've just found it really hard to resource the other wards, like to walk around, because I feel as if I haven't had time to even drag somebody from another ward to say, 'Hey, what resources have you got up here, can you show me...'. I feel as if I would have to go and find somebody and capture them and say, 'This is what our ward is doing, and can you help me find this on the ward, please'. I'm finding that difficult.

It is evident from these comments that trying to involve other units in the same hospital is a problem for nurses whose PAR project is an adjunct to, rather than part of, their recognised work role. Nurses working in large academic settings equally often it difficult to keep abreast of their colleagues or inform them of their own research. Community nurses are often the most isolated and have no opportunity to tell the detail of their practice much less communicate their research. In my travels I have heard stories of the isolation of nursing research and researchers repeated constantly.

Ethical issues and protocols

Ethics committees are set up to examine technical, medical research. They may have a panel to judge the technical aspect of the proposal prior to the committee or it may be done in the committee by scientists and lay people who have been taught what to expect in a research proposal. Nurses who are interested in qualitative research or PAR generally have more difficulty obtaining consent from ethics committees because they present their material in a form which is different from what the members of the committee expect and understand as good scientific research.

Nurses have taken a number of different stances to deal with ethics committees and there are no right answers. One problem in writing a proposal which tries to meet the presumed expectations of the ethics committee is that if we are not careful we may find that the research that is approved is not the research we want to do. Alternatively, we may actually have our proposal assessed by someone who understands qualitative research and wonders about us if we use categories like 'reliability'. Nurses who attempt to be true to the language and structure of a qualitative project, and educate the committee, may find that they are disadvantaged and do not receive approval.

I have found that the middle road is the safer. I use as many categories as I can which are common to all research and as many headings as possible to clarify meaning. At the same time I try to stay consistent with the theoretical and methodological implications of the chosen research design. The headings which I generally use are as follows:

Elements of a research protocol

- Research title
- Principal investigators
- Research objective
- Research questions
- Estimated length of project

- Financial support
- Resource implications
- Institutional support
- Historical background and rationale
- Literature review
- Theoretical perspective
- Significance of the project
- Methodology
- Research design
    Research participant selection and size
    Recruitment process
    Data collection strategies
    Data management
    Data analysis
    Reporting of research
- Ethical issues
    Participant information form
    Informed consent form.

This outline provides a guide for projects where an official ethics form is not provided. It organises some of the information necessary to describe a research project in an application to an institutional ethics committee.

Ethical considerations

It is important for any research to acknowledge the rights and responsibilities of the participants and others who may inadvertently be affected by it. This involves thinking about whether it is necessary to inform others of the aims and methods of the proposed research and gain their permission. When we are developing proposals for participatory research participants there is a series of questions we should ask ourselves that are fundamentally directed at examining research ethics.

With whom am I working and how are rights being safeguarded?

This is a general question aimed at identifying the ethical components of research with human subjects be they nursing colleagues, other staff, patients or families. From this general question we are led to specific questions of consent, confidentiality, and so forth.

Informed consent

How is informed consent being arranged?

A common mistake made by novice researchers is to ignore the need to explain the actual processes by which informed consent is to obtained from patients or clients taking part. It is not sufficient to say, 'I will obtain informed consent'. The process will involve a form of written explanation of the research aims, processes and consequences to the participant which is generally supported by an initial discussion. In many cases informed consent is obtained a couple of days after the explanation has been given so that the participant has a cooling off period. This cooling off period provides time for the person to think through the consequences of what is proposed, away from any enthusiastic or coercive activities on behalf of the researcher. It gives them an opportunity to seek advice from others if they feel that will help them make an informed decision, and it provides time for them to think of any other questions they would like to have answered before they sign a consent form.

Confidentiality

How am I to protect the rights of those involved or affected
in terms of privacy, confidentiality and discretion?

Participatory research means that the participants are known to each other and this raises questions of protection of privacy and confidentiality.

As a parenthesis I want to mention here the issue of anonymity. Many novice researchers think that they are addressing anonymity by the use of code names. No one is anonymous if his or her identity is traceable either by the demographic data the research has or because that person originally had a name before it was coded. Anonymity is only preserved in large studies when questionnaires are distributed which do not require identifying data or the nature of the sample size means that any individual cannot be identified through the categories of information collected.

In participatory research a more important issue is the maintenance of confidentiality. Most funding bodies follow the guidelines for data collection and handling which are set out by the major government funders of research. These guidelines generally require details about when, where and how the names of participants are to be replaced by codes; where and how confidential material is stored and the length of storage time; the handling of audio and video tapes, computer disks and other forms of recording; and who will have access to the data and under what conditions. Information about access should deal not only with the research team but with secretarial or administrative staff who may handle very sensitive data about people's lives and by chance recognise a name such as a relative's neighbor or a trades person. It is common practice to require temporary typing staff to sign a form agreeing to keep confidential any information they might hear or read in the course of the job.

Coercion

Do the participants have free choice about
their involvement in the project?

It is important in any form of research that participants have free choice about whether they wish to be involved or not. This is not another part of the informed consent issue. Free choice relates to the conditions under which the participant is both informed and gives consent, and the extent to which the right to withdraw at any time without consequences, is protected. When people are to be asked to participate in the process of speaking to, being watched by, or having their documentation accessed by a researcher, it is vital that the researcher, or an independent person, conducts the recruiting carefully according to the approved ethical principles. Although permission is required for access to staff or patients or clients for research from managers and responsible health professionals, they may be an inappropriate choice to do the active recruiting because of their position. It is important that people don't agree to participate because they fear some retribution or unpleasant consequence if they refuse or withdraw. It is essential that a refusal to participate or a withdrawal is treated with respect and without prejudice to the individual in any form.

Potential harm to participants

Is there any potential harm to participants
and how is that being addressed?

In research ethics the issue of potential harm has generally been thought of in terms of surgical procedures, drug trials or double blind clinical trials, where the person is either subject to an experimental procedure, or access to a procedure is withheld until it has been assessed. In participatory projects which are focused on understanding and changing procedures, protocols and practices, nurses need to question seriously whether their activities may harm anyone. Generally nurses are very sensitive to this issue and manage it well, but it needs to be detailed in a proposal for an ethics committee.

Something that is often neglected is the acknowledgment that the interview method can also do harm if the discussion brings unresolved issues to the surface or revisits upsetting experiences. Although well conducted interviews may affirm a person's sense of self-worth, be cathartic or validate their ideas and experiences, there is always the risk that re-living distressing experiences may cause real damage.

In situations where emotional harm is an obvious danger, such as interviewing people who have a psychiatric history, there are a number of safeguards that need to be established. One protocol, which I believe manages this well, asks the interviewee to identify a person who is familiar with their situation and whom they trust to be with them through this process. This support person may also attend the interview if that is the interviewee's wish or be present in the same building—ready and available at any time. At the conclusion of the interview the support person will debrief the interviewee in a comfortable environment of their own choosing. The support person will also have previously agreed to be available to provide up to three follow-up counselling sessions if that is seen as valuable by the interviewee. Protocols of this nature take seriously the potential for the discussion of disturbing events to destabilise an individual. In the same way, nurses who may be interviewed about traumatic events should have a designated counsellor or appropriate person made available to them if they think that they need to debrief in a professional context. Debriefing of participants after an interview or focus group should be organised as part of the ethical process of preventing harm to participants. Nurses engaged in PAR and other similar methods will debrief as part of the reflection process.

Participants in a research group who are investigating an episode, in their own practice or experience, which is traumatic or which distresses them can provide ongoing debriefing and support for each other—the tissue box research meeting! However it needs to be accepted that sometimes an individual's experience may be such that he or she needs to withdraw from membership of the research team without being made to feel that they have let the team down.

Deception

Are we practising deception, and is that justifiable?

Deception is an issue when researchers are investigating the attitudes or actions of a group of people and believe that if they reveal the real agenda the subjects will act differently and 'bias' the research. Because they are focused on the experience, attitudes and practice of the participants, participatory research designs generally do not have this problem. This also fits in with a research view which suggests that whatever information is collected about people at a particular time may not necessarily be representative of the person's normal view or practice, or that the situation of being watched or questioned or 'researched' may not influence the responses except in the short term. To understand this better, think what it is like to have visitors come and stay in your house for a time. You may be able to keep up appearances in the short term, but after a few days the laundry reverts to its untidy state or you begin to yell at the kids again, and the facade crumbles under the pressure of your own habitual responses. Participatory researchers are concerned with unpicking their own habitual patterns and responses, which emerge over time. So deception is rarely possible or necessary in these forms of research.

Privileged access to data

Does anyone have privileged access to the data or the findings?

Research which has the potential to uncover habits and practices which may not conform with the mission statement of an agency, or with the agency produced protocols, may concern administrators. They may be concerned that the area under their jurisdiction is to be revealed as functioning differently from their reports. Other groups may wish to have access to research data to show anomalies which support their industrial claims. Other people again are worried about what might have been said about themselves or about someone they care about. There are a variety of reasons why some people may endeavour to establish their credentials for having privileged access to research data. How this issue is to be dealt with needs to be spelt out in an ethical protocol. In participatory research it may mean that participants deal with sensitive data at the same time and that no one participant has prior access.

Benefits to participants and agency

Who will benefit from this project and how?

Most of what is written on an ethics committee application is concerned with how the researchers intend to safeguard the rights of others. However there is also a need to state the benefits to the participants from the research. These may be tangible like money or a special service. They may also be less tangible but equally beneficial: new knowledge or a sympathetic and interested audience. It is important not to overrate these benefits.

The benefits to the institution are equally important. In a time of pressure for more productivity from fewer staff, many managers are reluctant to have too many research projects in their area if they cannot see clear benefits. Another concern is the protection of vulnerable clients from being 'over-researched'.

Obligations and responsibilities

What are the responsibilities and obligations
of the research participants or the agency?

The obligations and responsibilities of the participants need to be explained. They need to be clear if it is necessary that they complete a questionnaire, agree to be interviewed, agree to keep information confidential, agree to attend a number of focus groups, or agree to follow a proposed action and report on the consequences. The participants need to understand exactly what they are being asked to do in the research.

Likewise, it is important that any institution or agency understands that they are giving permission for staff to be interviewed, or attend meetings, or to use existing material resources.

Any project which requires action involving the recipients of nursing care needs to be authorised by an institutional ethics committee. At times I have found that nurses want to conduct a preliminary single interview with children or their parents to provide some basic information. If this constitutes the introductory pilot phase of research and can be subsumed in what is considered normal nursing practice then it should not require ethics committee approval. As most nursing PAR is concerned with the practice of nurses and is intimately related to what fits into the realm of normal nursing practice it may not need approval. However it will still need unit management support, and approval from a nursing research management group or similar entity. For example, a PAR group who have designed a new admission assessment tool may wish to trial it with some of their patients. As the use of a standardised assessment tool for recording patient information is normal nursing practice, ethics committee consent is not necessary, although management consent is.

However if patients and families are to be interviewed in a way that goes beyond the limits of common nursing practice, the project will require ethics committee approval. If other nurses beyond the research group are to be asked to participate then they will still require a letter explaining the research and in some instances may be asked to sign a consent form which meets the ethics committee standards.

Research participant information form

Any form devised for patient, family or research participant information needs to include the following information in plain English:

- Research title
- The aim of the research recruitment process
- The full extent of the involvement of the research participants —include possible side effects, consequences, expectations, etc.
- Methods of data collection and management
- Freedom of consent and processes of withdrawal from the research
- Data and reporting access
- Direct benefits to the participants
- Funding arrangements
- Researchers' institutional identification and contact numbers
- Process of consent giving.

Data collection revisited

I have worked with nurses to identify which data collection methods they themselves found most congruent with their own skills and interests. Essentially these methods used the nursing skills of observation, oral communication, analysis of recorded information and responsive action. I have listed a number of these methods in the box but will comment further on those that are used most extensively by nurses and those which we have developed for particular use in participatory projects.

Observation and recording
Statistics
Charts
Participant observation
Journals
Diaries and logs
Portfolios
Case notes
Photos, audio tapes and videos
Conferences
Minutes and appointment books

Asking questions
Semi-structured interview—open ended
Focused conversations
Collaborative dialogues
In-depth interviewing
Questionnaires
Surveys

Reading
Historical documents
Literature review
Policy document analysis
Memorandum, newsletters, reports
Medical records
Budgets
Rosters and files
Legislation and regulations

Deciding to explore methods which build on existing nursing skills was a learning process. Initially we all began by assuming that we would collect information in conventional ways and, since for most nurses, their experience of research with human subjects involved measuring and collecting statistical data or participating in endless questionnaires, that was what they wanted to do.

Collecting statistics

Statistics are very valuable when you want to explore whether a problem is a recurrent one or experienced by a large number of people. Nurses interested in evaluating and improving the effectiveness of their discharge education devised information sheets and their colleagues were required to fill in details whenever they encountered another episode of the problem under consideration. However the group met some problems and it is instructive to see how these novices learned about statistical data in the process of doing it.

The first sheets were simple. They asked for certain information, such as how many times families phoned with questions after discharge, but the nurses discovered that these figures were of limited value. They didn't provide information on what the relatives were phoning about. The next data collection sheet was more comprehensive. A series of categories—pain, medication, wound care, etc.—provided more information but still did not bring out what kind of information the relatives were seeking in these categories. A further column was added for examples of questions to be noted. The documentation was becoming more time consuming and the nurses found their colleagues less zealous in their record keeping. The nurses had to decide how useful intermittent recording was to their project. In other words, how large did their sample need to be and how consistently had the data to be recorded to be considered valid.

A further examination of the information collected for later analysis of this group's plan indicated other problems. The action plan involved the trial of a new discharge information process and information sheet for a particular medical condition which appeared to be the source of concern for the relatives of discharged persons. Maintenance of the data collection process was intended to demonstrate the effectiveness of the new strategy. However the data collection sheet now captured all the information about the number of phone calls and the questions asked by the patient's carers but this information was not contextualised. The available statistics needed to be assessed against the monthly population of patients on the ward who had the medical condition in question.

In this case the researchers could have moved in at any time and insisted that they design an appropriate tool, however the experience was not only about discharge education but also about learning research by doing it—discovery learning of the kind that demonstrated the uses and misuses of data collection. The nurses who worked on this project became very clear about how they would need to collect statistical data in future and now understood the complexities and relationships of research design.

Questionnaires

My experience of working with novice researchers has illustrated time and again that the questionnaire is the research tool which is the most popular and the least understood. It is understandable when questionnaires appear to be the most common tool for information gathering in health research. A good questionnaire is an excellent way to collect consistent information from a large number of people, however questionnaires are not always the best method for novices and questionnaire development is considered a very difficult task by seasoned researchers. On one project which used both a survey questionnaire and in-depth interviews I asked a senior medical researcher with an international reputation if I could have permission to use one section of his questionnaire as it was reliable and valid and had been used and tested for years. He was very generous in allowing me to use his work but warned me that he was still very unhappy with it after twelve years and hoped I might be able to point out ways it could be improved.

Working with both inexperienced and experienced researchers in questionnaire development has made me sensitive to the problem of attempting to make the questionnaire do more than is appropriate. One PAR group I was involved with decided to develop a short questionnaire of no more than ten questions. The group had a week to consider what should be included. Every member did this very zealously and when we met again each had at least thirty questions to contribute. As one nurse commented:

Well it was amazing really! We all wanted our own questions to be included and even when you pointed out that many of the questions were concerned with the same thing we all wanted our wording put in...I know I did because I had sat up for two hours working on mine, I guess the others had too...and another thing was that even though I had worked hard—you know we had talked about open and closed questions and I had tried to do that—well we still didn't get them right...and you were right we did want to ask them everything under the sun and it did sound like a pass[or] fail test...and it was very biased, and well it was all much harder to do than I had thought.

This experience was repeated when I was working with an experienced bio-statistician whose research interests were similar to the topic the group was pursuing. She also wanted to add in parts to the questionnaire which related more to her interests than ours. Fortunately we did a trial of the questionnaire and it became evident that, as a tool, it was too lengthy, somewhat repetitious and attempting to cover too much material. This is an important lesson. If experienced researchers are keen to trial questionnaires then novice researchers need to do likewise. Developing effective questionnaires is the first step. Being able to analyse them is just as important. One group member wrote about the issues in development and analysis like this:

How To Develop A Headache Without Really Trying

If anyone ever thinks, 'Aha, we will do a questionnaire', *forget it.* After constructing the questionnaire and getting the responses back, then the next problem we faced was what to do with the information and how to write it up…We also did not realise how difficult it would be to correlate the data that was collected from the questionnaires or what the responses that we received meant to us as a group…about our own decision making processes.

For the purposes of some projects it may be possible to develop some simple forms of analysing the data using basic tools like graphs, bar charts or listing the number of respondents who replied either 'yes' or 'no' to basic questions. However if it is necessary for the information to be reliable and valid then more rigorous forms of analysis may be necessary. These may involve specific statistical tests so it is important for novice researchers to be mentored by experienced survey researchers to have access to adequate resources. Qualitative questionnaires also require rigor in analysis through forms of coding and indexing and at times through sophisticated theorising. Experienced researchers are essential guides at this stage in the research.

Interviews with a difference

There are many informative books on research interviewing. Most of them assume a position that the researcher is interviewing to obtain information from the interviewee and not to bring their own interests and assumptions to bear on the topic. Reflexive interviewing assumes that the interviewee participant is engaged in a negotiated, meaning making exercise in collaboration with the interviewer and is able to participate in the decision making processes about how information is collected and how it is used. In this section I want to write about two methods of reflexive interviewing—focused conversations and collaborative dialogues. Collaborative dialogues more truly reflect the participatory process of reciprocity and negotiated meaning making. However we have found that focused conversations provide colleagues with another enjoyable way of collaborating to explore their knowledge and practices.

Focused conversations

During 1992 I did some collaborative supervision work with Darrell Caulley, a methodologist from the school of education at La Trobe University. He spoke eloquently of the dilemmas of questionnaire construction and of the value of 'conversations with a purpose' to elicit information. He envisaged this use of conversation as an adjunct to participant observation. His descriptions of it fitted well with an idea I had been developing to help nurses gain information from their colleagues particularly during the reconnaissance stage. I had named the method 'focused conversations' and so began to develop them further and trial them with a group of nurses who wanted to find out the experiences and ideas of their colleagues in relation to their research topic.

As we began to work with focused conversations the initial concern of the nurses was that they would be unable to get the kind of information that was helpful. I offered to interview group members for seven minutes on the topic of concern to determine whether an experienced research interviewer could obtain useful information. I began with the question, 'Tell me your experience of [research topic] on the unit over the last three years?' With a few further judicious probes the nurses found themselves speaking about their ideas, experiences and attitudes. The other nurses were amazed at the amount of valuable information which emerged—information they would never have considered putting in a questionnaire—and information at a depth that is only possible when people have the time to explain their position.

The next task was for the nurses to use the method themselves. We practised with each other, taping the focused conversations for these novice interviewers to listen to. The nurses found it difficult to allow a time of silence for the other person to collect their thoughts and continue. The tendency was to rush in and provide a number of alternative answers—'Do you think that was because of this [provide a reason] or this [provide another reason] or this?'

The nurses also found themselves tempted to put in their own opinions or to take the conversation off on another track in their desire to cover as much ground as possible. A further challenge was learning to concentrate on what the other person was saying, and provide a probe to pursue that idea further, rather than focus on what oneself, the interviewer, wanted to say next. Through this encouragement and the opportunity to hear the tapes and recognise their own errors, the group of nurses rapidly learnt to ask an open question and then relax and listen. They realised that this was not an oral questionnaire but an opportunity to be still and really hear the interesting and valuable things their colleagues had to tell.

The focused conversations provided a lot of information in a short time. One group of five nurses had a focused conversation with six nurses each during a week. An information sheet detailing the research topic and the conversation process was distributed through the ward at the start of the week. At the start of each focused conversation the interviewing nurse explained the project and outlined the ethical considerations and the measures being taken to deal with confidentiality. If the interviewee agreed to participate in a focused conversation then the two went into the office and signed a consent form before the interview. The consent process took about three minutes and each focused conversation lasted between seven and ten minutes. Every conversation was taped on a mini dictaphone which was transcribed by the medical secretary. At the end of the week there were over five hours of tape recorded data and transcripts representing the ideas, attitudes and experiences of thirty-five nurses, including the research group.

As the group was not experienced at data analysis, we worked on the transcripts together. We sat around a large table listening to the tape and reading through the transcripts. We listed the issues and themes as they emerged on a large piece of paper and flagged specific examples as we encountered them. By marking each theme or issue as it came up again we were able to document those issues seen as important by a large number of people in the group. By listening to the tape we were also able to identify those matters which people felt strongly about by noting the passion and emphasis in their voices.

We also discovered some things which were not commonly spoken about but which when mentioned immediately 'rang bells' for each group member. As one remarked:

That's interesting...she's the only one to mention that but it sure rings bells with me [noises of assent from group]...That happens often but we just don't talk about it do we? [agreement from group members]...See we all think that is important but none of us said it in our focused conversation.

The group members agreed and so we revisited the transcripts to locate those things that may have been overlooked in the first reading, things which were suppressed because nurses have not been encouraged to speak about them or expect to find them in the data.

Initially the nurses found it hard to categorise the information and to agree on appropriate labels. After some initial work a review of the categories which had emerged in the literature helped group members organise the material. Over time they became quite skilled at identifying and structuring the data.

Collaborative dialogues

Another form of interview which fitted with the aim of reciprocity in the praxis was a process we named collaborative dialogues. These dialogues were designed to elicit information from the person being interviewed while at the same time conveying information back and challenging taken for granted assumptions. The method was used in contexts where a collaborative relationship had been developed with staff who were prepared to investigate particular issues further. For example, when nursing staff talked at length about the way that medical or administrative practices limited their own practice, we would work together to explore how this occurred and in what ways the actions of the nurses contributed to the continuance of the situation. We also examined our own research practices and sought to disclose the taken for granted assumptions in them along with those practices which we complained about but maintained through our own actions. These dialogues involved two or more researchers and one or more research participants. Using an agreed outline of key questions, we would explore together, and challenge each other, so as to arrive at a better understanding of the shape of the issue under investigation.

Journalling is used extensively by nurses as a form of data collection for analysis and reflection in participatory projects (see Oberg 1990). However, as I conceive of it as a reflective research method in its own right I have devoted Chapter 7 to a more extensive exploration of keeping a journal.

After the action has been implemented and the data collected and analysed the action research process requires that the participants engage in critical reflection. This process will be explored further in Chapter 6.

6. Reflection and the research report

Critical reflection is an interesting and powerful thing. It can send us on an investigation which can change our lives by leading us to further discoveries about ourselves and others. A fascinating example of critical reflection is the story of the discovery of the planet Neptune. When Uranus was discovered in 1781 by Herschel it was considered that humanity had discovered the end of the solar system and all that was left to do was to plot the orbits of the planets. This view persisted although the task of plotting the orbit of Uranus caused some difficulty. It seemed that it wandered off course in a way that defied any known explanation. In 1846, independently of each other, a French astronomer Le Verrier and an English mathematician Adams engaged in some critical thinking and came to the conclusion that the calculations they were amassing must mean that there was another planet in the close vicinity of Uranus whose planetary mass was pulling Uranus out of orbit. As no further planet was discernible each used their theoretical technical knowledge to work out the orbit of this unseen planet. With these calculations two German astronomers, Galle and d'Arrest, knew where to look in the sky with their telescopes and discovered Neptune. On this basis further mathematical calculations were made by Lowell, which finally led to the discovery of barely visible Pluto by Tombaugh in 1930 (Ridpath 1985).

This story fascinates me because it not only demonstrates the power of unblinkered critical thought followed by systematic and disciplined knowledge and action, but it also demonstrates the lucky element in the midst of the so called hard sciences—the imagination of the scientist at work asking new questions and finding new answers.

Asking nurses to reflect critically on their own research experience can show how they can unpick their assumptions and habitual ways of acting. One nurse who had been involved in PAR

projects for nearly four years reflected on his early understandings
of the research process:

Initially...we didn't really understand the action research process, it
was really only at the end when we looked back and reflected on it,
we realised that we were starting to understand the process.

Not only did the group members not really understand the
process until they had joined in using it for a period of time, but
they also had difficulty recognising what they had achieved. They
realised that they had confused research with education:

Our initial thing was, we didn't really achieve anything...our idea of
achieving something was to set up a program to educate people. But
in fact we felt, on reflection, again, we...achieved something, by
learning a lot more about the issues of resuscitation. Like one of the
questions we were first asked, 'Well, what issue to you want to look
at in regards to resuscitation?' and we sort of said 'Oh, we just want
to look at the whole lot'. And it was only after sort of talking about our
experiences and sort of sifting through those, and saying, 'Well, these
issues just continually arise', and we said, 'Well, why do these issues
continually arise?' Things such as, you know, 'Why do nursing staff
sort of always feel like on the outer?', and 'Why aren't parents
involved?' and 'What's the most important thing about resuscitation
to the nurses, and to the doctors?' and whatever. So we looked at
that over a period of time, and...I mean I feel that we gained something
out of it, and we produced a paper.

In this account we can see that the nurse was able not only to
identify a process of change in the understanding of the participants
about their chosen topic but also in the understanding they had of
the process of PAR. This process of change moved from a medically
oriented approach to a clearer nursing focus:

When we first started the majority of the group wanted to look at
things like, 'How many compressions that you do on the heart for
different age groups', so for an infant, whether it be 120 or 140 per
minute, and for an adult, you know, 60 to 80. How many breaths you
do, and what sort of drugs you give, and they were the sort of...the
anxiety related things, but they were all very medical related.

Through a process of reflection these nurses were able to see
that the questions they were concerned with were medically-
oriented knowledge questions. They realised that an improvement
in knowledge would help improve staff confidence but as they
discussed their experiences further they discovered that staff often

had the appropriate knowledge but were anxious because other aspects of the topic were not being acknowledged. They found that they needed to examine different questions:

But we sort of started to say, 'Well, hang on, why are the parents locked out?' 'What happens to us as nurses, after the "resus"?'. 'Who sits down and says, "You did a good job", or "You did a bad job", and "These are the reasons why we thought it [the resuscitation] was good or bad"? Why is it that people say, if the kid survives it 'it was a good resus.' and if the kid dies, 'It was a bad resus'?...Eventually we looked at what we do as nurses for the resuscitation.

This reflection process set the group on a divergent and important track in their research. They began to see that various staff carried out different roles and that new staff would always be assisted in the mechanical aspects of resuscitation. They also perceived that what was generally assumed, and yet often missed, was the orientation of new staff to their roles in checking equipment and checking the status of the child at the start of each shift. Then they were emboldened to think about how to deal with the parents of the child or other parents who may be present in the unit visiting their own children and becoming distressed by the arrest. Finally they were led to establish an evaluative debriefing session for the staff involved. One nurse described this change as the establishment of a formal procedure to orient new staff:

Instead of saying, 'Go off over to the store and do this "resus" course', we would tell them to grab one person on the ward who's fairly experienced, and just go through a resuscitation, and [we'd] say, 'Look, you're not going to get into trouble for not knowing your compressions, because someone will get in and shoulder you out of the way and do that for you'. But if you have got the kid by the bed, and your suction's not going, people are going to say, 'Well why wasn't that going?', 'Why wasn't your oxygen connected?' and the things you really need to know are whether you move the child and what's happening with mum and dad.

Despite the response from staff and the experience that the action plans of this new approach were more effective, this nurse was also able to reflect on how this nursing research still felt:

Very wishy washy...compared with what we've done for years...to look at the physical side of things.

Although the nurses were able to perceive the effect of medical dominance in the way they structured their early questions and action plans, they still devalued their own research practices in comparison with some mythical form of 'medical' research. It takes time and support to unpick individual habitual ways of being, which is why group reflection and participatory processes are valuable.

Group reflection

Group reflection requires the participants to embark collaboratively on a process of critical reflection which enables them to stand back from the action and analysis to review the reconnaissance, action plan and data collection strategies in the light of what they have learned and how the situation has changed.

Wadsworth (1991) suggests that this process means that PARs come to understand the practical and ethical implications or the values and effects of their inquiry:

- the effects of their raising some questions and not others
- the effects of their involving some people in the process (or even apparently only one) and not others
- the effects of their observing some phenomena and not others
- the effects of their making this sense of it and not alternative senses (Wadsworth 1991:3).

The process of reflection asks the group to disentangle their taken for granted assumptions and think creatively about the structures and limitations of their practice.

A group of nurses were concerned that children from non English speaking backgrounds were not eating well in hospital because the food they were being offered was culturally inappropriate. Initially they discussed this issue in relation to the hospital dietary kitchen. Through the critical reflection process they discovered that their own nursing practices in relation to diet could be reviewed. They identified the Anglo-Australian assumptions inherent in their practice, which assumed that children with gastroenteritis from any cultural group would respond to a diet based on toast. This insight sent them to speak to the dietitian and then to workers from migrant health resources. One nurse reported to the group the information which she had obtained regarding suitable foods for children with 'gastro':

The Sri Lankans use water and sugar ['their water is fairly saline anyway', she said] or boiled rice left watery. The Lebanese use bread and yoghurt. Asian people roast rice and mix it with water...Italians mix boiled rice with parmesan cheese, but [she'd] never seen it...Central Americans' diet is based on beans and lentils, bean curd, etc...Rice is fairly universal. Central American countries grow corn, [e.g. tacos], beans, etc.

This group was able to recognise that if they wished to help non English speaking families with children who had digestive problems, they not only needed to get an interpreter to explain the dietary needs, they also needed to make sure the proposed diet was familiar and acceptable to the family. By reflecting critically on their own practices they were able to identify ways in which their assumptions about toast as a regular gastroenteritis diet had been challenged and they were able to develop action plans to inform other staff and change the inappropriate habitual advice that was being given.

Facilitating the group reflection process

In order for nurses to work through a reflective process I have found that the following guidelines are helpful. I usually ask the group to re-state briefly their action plan and the chosen method of data collection. This reminds them of what the issue of concern is and the how they had decided to act and monitor their action.

What happened when you put your plan into action?

An ability to recount the actual events which occurred as a result of the implementation of an action plan is essential as a basis for further examination of the complexities of the situation.

Shifts and rosters mean that many PAR groups are small and so are not representative of the staff in a particular unit. A common concern for many of these groups at the start is to determine whether their experience is shared by most staff. For some groups this need to examine the extent of the problem as perceived by others becomes their first action plan and data collection stage. For example, one group wrote:

Action Plan 1—Do other staff share our concern?
After the major issues were decided we then had to plan the way we thought best to gain other staff members' feelings on the issue. We needed to determine what were the major issues for them, and whether they concurred with our thoughts.

This group had decided to use a questionnaire as their data collection strategy. They reported back to a larger research steering group meeting their group reflection:

We decided to formulate a questionnaire as we thought this would be an efficient way of getting written information from the staff. However this was far from true. We originally sent questionnaires to fifteen anonymous randomly selected nursing staff. We looked at the roster list and randomly selected every person and sent a questionnaire.

What were the consequences of your action?

This group recounted their disappointment and anger at the poor response to their questionnaire. During the ensuing discussion on the reasons for poor response rates, members admitted that they also were guilty of ignoring questionnaires or notices. The nurses unravelled the history of this poor response rate. They observed that their experience of being asked to participate in activities which didn't eventuate or were considered a waste of time, along with their experience of responding to surveys which 'went nowhere as far as we were concerned', had led them to ignore such requests as much as possible. It was possible to trace a form of passive resistance which occurred as a result of having initially been enthusiastic and conscientious only to receive no discernible benefits to themselves 'only more time-wasting when we don't have time!'

Dealing with the question of what consequences there are alerts the group members to the fact that any social research with an action component has repercussions, which are either intended or unintended, expected or unexpected.

Group members can learn important lessons from reflection about the conduct of clinical research within nursing culture. For one group this part of the process enabled them to find out that their plan was being talked about and adopted by other nurses on the unit. The other staff had heard about it through the unit meeting, seen it in action and thought that they would use the procedure too. This was unintended. The other staff did not have the background to the problem so they were not implementing the plan systematically or collecting the relevant data. The nurses in the PAR group decided that as others must think it was a good idea they had better change their initial idea, which was to trial it only with a small group, and involve a lot more staff in the trial.

For another group the unexpected consequences related to their data collection strategy:

The writing up of the information gained in order for it to be relevant to the problems identified also presented us with a problem. In fact it became clear that our questionnaire was somewhat biased in the questions that were asked, and that the issues that were identified by the initial group members were not necessarily seen as the main issues by everyone!

Without this time of stopping the action and reflecting upon its consequences there is a real danger of problems not being identified and redressed in the replan stage of problem reformulation.

What feedback did you receive from other people?

PAR is structured on the assumption that people in a given situation have a good understanding of the needs of their given situation and are able to help each other. As one group reported:

When we went to the broader PAR community and told them our problems about getting responses from our sample, we were asked why we did not include all nursing staff, given that all staff were affected and the sampling was too small. This prompted us to reconsider our action plan and send the questionnaire out to all staff. Even then we discovered at a later meeting that not all staff had received a questionnaire, including the charge nurse.

How did your action affect yourself and others?

Actions conducted in the social world can affect both the research participants and others with whom they are involved. These questions remind us of the ethical dimension, which must be constantly monitored in this form of research. One group realised the effect on the participants and on others of their inadequate communication strategy.

At this time H was feeling despondent as there were few replies and they were all coming to her rather than the group members. It became apparent that staff saw it as H's project rather than a group concern. When we looked at what information we gave staff about the group, we had referred to ourselves as an action research group rather than inform staff of the specific participants in the project. There were also at that time six other action research projects in progress in the unit, all calling themselves the action research group.

This account demonstrates that careful reflection can reveal exactly how language affects understanding.

The problem of who 'owns' the group was one which many groups encountered when the group was identified with an enthusiastic or senior person rather than seen as a collaborative exercise. It was interesting to chart in the research notes when a group moved from being 'owned' by a person and became 'our' group.

An opportunity for group members to reflect on how their research was affecting them led one nurse to report:

[The research has] been good...in a lot of regards from the point of view that it's opened our eyes to a lot of things on the ward. I mean a simple thing like...why weren't nurses using interpreters...and since the group being started I've just noticed that the majority of the nursing staff now just don't hesitate to ring up the interpreter, and get them to do the admission.

This nurse described a change in practice which showed that nurses valued their own work more and felt more confident to take initiatives. Another nurse gave an account of how being involved in examining cultural issues had sensitised them to other people's customs and tradition in a way that stopped them making eurocentric judgements:

We've been looking at other cultural issues as well. And one of the ones that we had some heated discussions over the other day was on circumcision. The Australian Medical Association is saying well, we've got to ban this, and...although none of us agreed with the female circumcision, we were all saying, 'Hang on, we're a multicultural society'. You know looking at it openly and [thinking] should we be saying, 'No, you can't do this', even though none of us agreed with it. We were just questioning that sort of attitude of stamp down, 'No, you can't do it'.

This is an interesting story because, although no one in the group actually wants to condone female circumcision, the nurses were also concerned that in a multicultural society a group of doctors could ban a practice without exploring the consequences. The research group discovered that their reflective practice meant that they were more open to thinking about the unthinkable in order to assess their own prejudices:

And now obviously some people said, 'Oh, it's barbaric' and all that sort of thing. Whereas, I think two years ago, it would have been all of us saying, 'No, it's just totally wrong, don't do it'. But some of us are now saying, 'Well, hang on', being a little bit more open. Not saying that we agree with it, but just saying, 'Well, there's always two sides to a story'. I think that's probably the extent of what I would call true research.

This nurse has linked an open and questioning attitude about a difficult and contentious ethical problem with the notion of doing research. She thinks that the attitudes of her peers have changed over the previous two years from a dogmatic answer to a research stance which wants to question and understand the situation— even in such an emotionally charged issue.

What problems did you encounter and how did you solve them?

Asking staff to articulate the problems they met helps them to understand their actions better and to develop more effective plans in future. Communication processes were an issue for one group who had worked on developing guidelines for the incoming registrars and residents. The guidelines explained the ward policies regarding discharge of elderly people with acute difficulties. These nurses were very concerned that the doctors did not inform them of proposed discharges in time to prepare the patients and their care givers adequately . The group found that the elderly people were often disoriented if rushed and needed time. The nurses were also concerned that families who came to collect a patient being discharged were both inconvenienced by, and often resentful at, having to wait for equipment or instruction. The unit manager set up a meeting with the new rotation of doctors to hand them with a copy of the guidelines and explain the processes of working effectively with the nursing staff. However only half the doctors attended. The nurses discussed their response:

We should have expected it...We were so enthusiastic and wanting to be positive. Anyway we decided that we would get them to listen to our side to explain how the procedures needed to work for everyone's good...So the unit manager and B and I went to see the medical 'supervisors' of the doctors and they agreed to set up a time for us to meet with the new registrars and residents each rotation when they are having their medical orientation...Now we have to see if it happens.

These nurses had expected that the new medical staff would be as interested at restructuring the communication processes as they were. They had not anticipated problems but, when they encountered them, they reflected on the usual situation and recognised that they had a great deal more invested in this than the doctors did. The doctors only saw their rotation as temporary whereas the permanent nursing staff were the ones to feel the wrath of patients and their families when communication broke down.

What resources did you use?

This question enables the group to be clear about resource issues. Many projects don't initially acknowledge the resources necessary for the action plans to be implemented. By asking the group to reflect on this practical issue they can plan more strategically in terms of future resource needs. As one nurse said:

> We were so used to just going to the cupboard and getting what we needed—this was in the good old days—but now with unit budgets being so tight then there isn't heaps of paper and envelopes and computer disks and tape recorders and all that stuff just lying around. You have to order it, and you have to say why you need it, particularly when we have shortages in other medical items.

When nurses learn to be clear about their resource needs they can be more effective as researchers.

What have you learnt as a result of this research?

The articulation of what participants have learnt about themselves, about their colleagues, about their language and about the situation is very important as a basis for making further informed decisions. One nurse has been involved in two PAR projects. At present the group she is involved with are concerned with focusing on ways to more effectively meet the emotional needs of children with serious cardiac conditions, particularly when these children are having painful procedures. She spoke to me about her changed nursing practice and assumptions in relation to the procedure of taking out a chest drain:

> Up until a couple of years ago...before you began working with PAR on the ward...when I was going to remove chest drains from a child I would ensure that I provided adequate pain relief prior to the removal. I suggested that the parents might like to stay, but not pushing them to as I was also telling them it's pretty ghastly [and that] they might like to wait outside. I then enlisted help from other staff. I'd have to negotiate with two people to help, and to hold a big child, perhaps a

fourth person. I would start enlisting early by saying, 'Would you be able to come and help me remove this chest drain in about five minutes?' because it was no easy task to get everyone at the same time. Then I'd explain the procedure to the child appropriate to its age…and here, and the expectation was that the child would wriggle and scream with two people holding it and two helping me…it was just the way it was and none of us like it but it had to be done.

In this account we can see that this nurse is explaining her previous practice and the assumptions which undergirded it. She went on to explain how she had changed:

Now first I explain to the mother or father and actively encourage them to stay. I ask them to focus on the child and try to distract him/her rather than concentrating on the procedure. If the child is old enough I will not talk while I am doing it but I will go ahead and do it. Sometimes the play specialist does the distraction if the mother isn't available or able to cope. With the child distracted you will only need two nurses [to do the procedure]. I try to move quickly and quietly through the procedure. and I don't teach [new staff] as I go. Before you'd teach someone all the time but now for new staff…I tell them what I will do before I start and tell them to watch. Then when it is all over we talk and answer any questions then.

I find the children are less stressed…they may still scream but then they look at mother for support and settle down quickly.

After explaining her changed practice this nurse spoke about other things she had learnt:

Before…whenever you put the screens up to do a procedure like this people used to put their head around the screens maybe six times during the procedure. People still try to, but I don't any more. Now I am always aware that when the screens are around I might be breaking the bonding or the concentration.

Overall by working on this issue of pain management, and using distraction for the removal of chest drains, and other things like the teaching and not interrupting others…it is all much better for the child and for us too. I didn't really think it would work but now we have less staff it takes less time and everyone is happy. It's good really.

This nurse has learnt how to use participatory research processes to improve her understanding and her practice.

In another unit the unit manager reflected on what had been learnt through the action research group on the unit.

On reflection...for the first time staff were exposed to the research process as an integral element of their own professional and personal development. By having staff raise the issues themselves and by taking action on those issues, I believe...empowered the nurses involved to make decisions about the nature of their work which would, in any other research methodology, have been denied.

The changes described by these nurses are minimal and may easily be passed over. The power of participatory research is that people reinforce each other's learning and support each other's practice.

During a recent consultancy process, many nurses who had been involved in PAR in different contexts came together to speak about their experiences. It was apparent that they had all been talking to each other—that the grapevine of research stories was flourishing. During some individual interviews nurses not only told their own stories—as we had expected; or the stories of their research group— which we had hoped for; but they also told stories which moved across the work of other groups, which they had heard about through their after hours networks. They then talked about the socio-political issues and effects—isolating the values inherent in the competing discourses and strategies so as to challenge policy and change practice. These nurses demonstrated consistently that they had learnt how to move from the micro politics of specific practices to the macro politics of larger ethical and socio-economic issues.

Replanning action

As PAR is a cyclical process which proceeds in small manageable loops, the reflection process generally leads on to another action plan to help the group members continue addressing their area of concern.

So the next questions can become, 'What will you do next?' followed by, 'How will you collect information about it?' and so the process continues.

One advantage of this cyclical process is that the movement in small loops enables the researchers to revisit and where necessary re-formulate the original question in the light of the evidence which has since emerged. This is particularly valuable for novice researchers engaged in research with people in social settings who may find themselves asking the wrong question or addressing the right question with the wrong method. Action research allows people to begin to learn the research process with a seemingly simple and practical question which matters to them.

One group began with what they perceived as a problem which would be easily fixed. A group member wrote:

We were greeted one night with a notice on the white board, stating:

Due to staff shortages on night duty—each person will have to do an increased amount of night duty in order to cover all the shifts. Put your name in the appropriate column stating your preference.

We were asked to give a preference on whether we would prefer to work six week days then two week nights or a month of nights and three months of days.

The notice presented to us was the first mention of increased night duty rotation. Instantly there were complaints. One RN especially was concerned, not only because of the increase in night duty, but because the staff affected by this decision were not being consulted before this decision was made.

At this point at least one staff member had recognised that the issue was not only related to the rostering process but also the manner by which the decision making process had occurred. However, although this concern was noted, the group planned their research with the expressed intention of improving the night duty roster. The low morale and high feeling associated with an increased disruption to their social lives meant that the nurses focused on the rotations as is evident in one nurse's account:

After being on night duty once again and finding out that I had to do it again in the near future, I decided to voice my opinion and distress about the increase in the night duty rotations that we were going to do. I, myself, had just returned from a month's annual leave, two weeks of which I spent overseas. It seemed that the ward morale was at an all time low despite many of us away on annual leave. The thought of any night duty made...us cringe—we simply hated doing it. Another nurse felt that it was disruptive to all aspects of her life and she couldn't spend valuable time with her husband. I don't sleep well at all when I am on night duty and spend the whole rotation deprived of sleep and normality. Another nurse simply cannot cope.

These nurses formed a group and negotiated with a clinical researcher to help them address their problem. The members expected that PAR would provide them with a process to solve their problem quickly. However they had not looked at the larger problem of hierarchically imposed decisions which impacted on people's social and emotional lives. As one RN wrote later to her colleagues:

Why Haven't I/We Fixed The Night Duty Rosters?

Like many of you, we thought that it was a relatively easy problem to solve, and would not take long. I mean, how long could it take to collect a few statistics about how people felt about the increase in the night duty rotation, and then put a few suggestions into practice with the charge nurse's guidance and authority. However, we were sadly mistaken about how long the whole process was to take, and this is one of the reasons why there has not yet been a solution to the problem.

I'm sure that if there was a quick way of fixing the roster problem that both the group and the charge nurse would have found it by now and the problem would be no more.

Theoretically a PAR group can continue as long as the participants see issues that they wish to pursue. However our experience has led us to structure groups with manageable time frames so that the participants do not become exhausted. There is only so much change that can be initiated and managed effectively within a ward at the one time and as PAR involves the participants in reflection on themselves there is also a limit to how much challenge to their ways of thinking and being busy staff can tolerate.

The setting up and development of PAR offered each nurse a sense of community and the privilege of being heard, which will have the most enduring effect. Rather than allowing ourselves to be seduced by our own research rhetoric—those arguments that talk of better conditions and happier nurses in the work place—we need to listen to the problems and concerns of nurses as they are raised and encountered in the work place itself.

Writing up

It is a challenge for nurses to learn the steps involved in systematic research, but it is often a greater hurdle when the research is finished and needs to be disseminated. As one nurse explained:

And there's not much confidence generally from nurses about starting from scratch writing a proposal, getting things like ethical approval, knowing where to get funding, doing the data collection and the data management, and we're talking about qualitative research here at the minute. And writing the report for dissemination, so that it is of a high standard, so that it can go out to journals for publication, etc. There is very, very little confidence at all.

One of the greatest difficulties we have encountered with clinical nurses is not a problem of getting motivated staff to do the research but the problem of getting them to write up their research for dissemination and publication. Writing research reports has not been part of the clinical nurse's role, and many find it difficult to know where to start. As researchers we have found that using headings and questions to format the report, and spending time talking to nurses about each part as they prepare it, has been effective but time-consuming. It has also been helpful to arrange for staff to work in a research unit consistently for a few days to help them concentrate. The nurses themselves express their satisfaction at this, but also their surprise at what hard work writing is. As one nurse explained:

You just can't get into it. When I came and worked over here for a few days with A, I mean, I found it actually quite draining, cause I would be here staring at the computer screen having to talk you know, the whole time. But it was really good. I got far more done.

The value of writing a report also lies in the selection and analysis of the data to be reported. Writing the story of the research in order to leave a decision trail means that the writer(s) revisit the research and can pinpoint what has been achieved. This is particularly useful with PAR where there are often slight, incremental changes which rapidly become taken for granted rituals and practices. One nurse clarified this for herself:

Because it had got to the stage when you think, 'Have I really achieved anything, have I really changed anything?' But when you actually see all the [research] stuff, and you're there for the day talking about it...you feel more relaxed, you get much more done and you see what you've achieved.

Some nurses do not want to be involved in writing up research. Others think they would like to see their name in print until they understand the commitment necessary. Whereas other nurses are willing to try but are very aware of their lack of knowledge:

Well, I think that there'd be very few staff, probably including myself, that could actually, off their own back, produce a proper research paper...I'd give it a good go, you know. I might think, 'Oh, this is pretty good', but I've just seen the way that people prepare a paper, and then get someone to go through it and they'll say, 'Oh, you can't do that...you can't do that...you can't do that'. It can be discouraging.

Nurses who had participated in graduate study were also aware that they might not have the ability to produce a research paper without considerable direction:

I mean, even having done tertiary study, it doesn't teach you how to actually produce a research paper. You can do a, you know, fifteen thousand word essay, and be quite nice, but not actually write it in research terms.

As researchers we have found that time spent with intensively motivated staff has been very valuable as they gain confidence and become a resource for others:

Once you've actually done a report…I mean, for me, 'cause I've done them before, I don't have to think about the fact that they're difficult to write [that is] until I work with people who've never written one and they get so stressed out about them. I think, 'Oh, yeah, I wouldn't have known how to write one, unless someone had shown me in the first place'.

PAR is perhaps more difficult to report than other forms of research. It is essentially a dynamic process, one which is not easily captured within the format of a research report. Unlike quantitative research which is well structured for reporting, PAR often appears to have opened up new horizons of thought and understanding which are multi-focused and multi-directional. There is a constant temptation on the part of the researcher to pursue these interesting questions into what seem to be side alleys, only to find out too late that they open out into wider fields filled with fascinating questions with great possibilities. For the quantitative researcher the task of choosing among many a profitable direction for research is struggled with, and achieved, before the research design is constructed. However, the qualitative researcher is tempted throughout the conduct of the research and indeed even at the writing up stage, to wander into new and potentially more fascinating paths. By acknowledging this difficulty we can begin to work creatively with the dynamic project material and the necessarily formal structure of a research report.

Researchers deliberately choose to engage in PAR because it is a process which openly acknowledges the subjective nature of issues, and, through reflection, places the actions and attitudes of the participants, and the process, under scrutiny. Through this process the habits and taken for granted attitudes of the participants emerge. The researchers, as participants, are not immune to the effects of examining their own attitudes and practices. Anxieties held by researchers about how much they themselves take for granted, and how ingrained this pattern of thinking is in their own capacity to engage in empowering PAR and about their ability to record the intricacy and subtlety of the research experience can complicate the project of writing up. The researcher is not only making selections from a wide range of profitable material for reporting, but choosing to record instances which demonstrate the habitual ways of thinking and acting which are common to all the research participants, including the researcher.

In order to provide some commentary upon the process I have addressed the issues in relation to a structure which covers the basics of what is expected.

STRUCTURE OF REPORT.

The research question

PAR begins with a problem or concern expressed as a question. However, as the research unfolds, further questions emerge which can often seem to be closer to the crux of the problem or concern. It is this process which Freire (1981) refers to as 'posing the problem', that is, the process of engaging in action and reflection evolves new questions. These new questions may become evident because the process of PAR has enabled more appropriate questions to emerge. Or they may emerge because the situation has changed through the progress of the research requiring a changed point of view which has, in turn, led to development of different questions.

How do we record this dynamic process of problem posing? The challenge is to be prepared to begin at the beginning and write about the original concern which instigated the research. This means resisting the enticement to rewrite the research based on the questions of current concern or interest. This sounds very basic, but, as PAR is a process which involves the participants in forms of critique, they soon become aware of the inadequacy of their initial questions, which do not deal with the complexities of the situation as they appear in hindsight.

The background to the problem

In PAR terms this can be seen as a recounting of the reconnaissance stage. It requires an account of the situation which prompted the initial concern. The account needs to spell out the historical conditions which shaped the situation along with an account of the hegemonic factors which continued to maintain the situation prior to the project.

The literature review

The literature review will include an overview of the current research on the research topic. As this will often be quantitative research which has framed its research question in a particular way, the action researchers will need to explain why they have made the decision to pursue PAR as a means of exploring the topic. In order to do this, the report will need to demonstrate the gaps in the current research which a PAR project will fill.

In a project for a thesis it is also common practice to theorise the deficiency in relation to the key theoretical concepts and issues upon which PAR is founded. Therefore issues such as the exercise of power, gender relations, discourse, cultural practices and social/ organisational relationships could be addressed theoretically as regards their relationship to the particular initial concern.

The research design

The purpose of the research design is to describe both the chosen methodology and the manner in which the research was set up and managed. The elaboration of the research design allows for descriptions of how decisions were made in relation to, or with, the participants, such as the general group membership, the numbers of participants, the methods of selecting participants, and other decisions such as meeting frequency, place and time. The account can provide reasons for the various decisions taken by the researcher and the participants demonstrating how these decisions were framed in response to the particular, and peculiar, conditions of the situation.

These changes have occurred in response to the process of the implementation of systematic action, collection and analysis of data, and critical reflection forming the basis of further problem-posing, action, analysis and reflection.

Findings and PAR process

The key issue turns on the need to represent the findings of the group in relation to the problems faced, while at the same time, representing the participant's progress through the action research process, depicting the issues uncovered and the strategies implemented.

This dilemma is resolved by some researchers through the format of a chronicle of the progress of the action research from the initial concern, through the changed action plans, implementation strategies and reflection. Other researchers choose to write about their action research thematically, based on the major theoretical themes which emerged as they worked with the material. Choices also have to be made concerning the form of the written account of the PAR, although this should reflect the manner of data analysis.

Concluding the report

Unlike a report of quantitative research which summarises the findings and when appropriate makes recommendations based on them, the concluding section of a PAR project may demonstrate creative ways of dealing with an issue. For example, it may provide an example of the power of collaborative action and reflection to provide new understanding of ethical or theoretical issues, which in turn can lead to changes in the situation. However, although the issues themselves may be readily generalisable, the action taken by the PAR group, while being informative and challenging, will not be generalisable because it is context specific, responding to the particular historical, social and political conditions of the situation researched. Therefore there may be no findings that can justify specific recommendations, unless simply that certain questions need to be addressed by particular groups and that PAR can provide a process which is suitable and relevant.

Writing about the reflective process

PAR as a reflective process provides all the participants with the opportunity to reflect not only upon the issues and actions that they have been immersed in but upon their use of the process. The final reflection upon the processes and decisions can be very illuminating for the participants and for the reader. This section of the research report can provide the reader with insight into why particular actions and decisions were made, how the meaning making process unfolded and how the participants dealt with their own doubts, dilemmas and disappointments when faced with their own 'unpicked' habits and attitudes.

7. Behind the research scene

Most research reports focus on what has been discovered by the researchers throughout the progress of the research. The emphasis is on the topic and what has been learnt in relation to the question or hypothesis of the researcher. Therefore the focus is on the unfolding drama which occurs center stage. The research method is justified but it is not common for mainstream research to allocate much space to the reporting of the activities of the 'behind the scenes' crew who make the play happen. In this section the emphasis is on what happens behind the scenes of a praxis research process— how decisions were made and what has been learnt in the process. To illustrate this I have chosen to highlight the developments which occurred in the pilot stage of a larger research project. This pilot stage was a collaborated project with Chris Walsh and the community mental health nurses located at Hutt, near Wellington in New Zealand.

Finding a research topic

Research begins with an idea; a research team begins with shared interests and complementary skills. This research project began with a merging of interests and an acknowledgment of the particular skills and knowledge that Chris and I had to offer each other in a research team.

I was in New Zealand on one of a number of visits as scholar-in-residence when I received an invitation to give a keynote address on the topic of nursing research at the 1993 National Psychiatric Nursing Conference. As I have a policy that I speak within my areas of expertise and use my current research, I was bothered about this invitation. I had done no research in the psychiatric area and to speak about research processes using my current research, which at that time was involved with child and family health in

Australia, would be very inappropriate to the New Zealand context and to psychiatric nursing. I was impressed with the psychiatric nurses I had met and was interested in working with some of them to develop a small research project which could provide material for my keynote address and make a contribution to the local scene. I had already met Chris Walsh, who had taken leave from her college teaching post to do an applied Master's degree in social research. She had been doing some relieving work as a community health nurse in the Hutt region and describes her experience:

Early in 1993 I took the opportunity to work in the community as a psychiatric nurse replacing staff members who were on leave. This was a huge relief to me as I had taken leave without pay from my job as a lecturer at Wellington Polytech to do post graduate studies at Victoria University. When the offer of this work was made I saw it as an opportunity not only to earn some money but also to revisit the practice area as a staff nurse, no mean feat after 4 years lecturing in nursing!

One of the first changes that I was aware I would encounter was the newly instituted Mental Health Act and the role of nurses working in the community as duly authorised officers (DAO). While I had some knowledge of the new Act I was uncertain how the changed provisions and procedures for assessment and treatment would impact on me as a relieving community psychiatric nurse. I was not a DAO and thought that I would be at a disadvantage in my nursing practice. When I mentioned this to various people they assured me that it would be OK and since I was only relieving others would be able to function in that capacity if necessary for the clients that I was looking after.

The experience of revisiting the practice area reassured me that I hadn't lost my touch as a psychiatric nurse and was able to strike up therapeutic relationships with clients fairly rapidly. More importantly I connected again with staff, some of whom I worked with some years ago, and felt part of a team that was sometimes under enormous pressure to work 'productively' in a health system that was, and is, more concerned with measuring outputs and cutting costs than with the realities of de-institutionalisation. I often felt it would be a useful exercise to take some of these politicians into some of the homes that I visited and see how long they could sustain their policies in the face of poor living conditions and lack of support for caregivers.

I have always felt that as psychiatric nurses we have failed to articulate our practice and that this has lead to a poor understanding of what it is that we do. Psychiatric nursing is a skilled and undervalued profession and psychiatric nurses need to rectify this by promoting their profession particularly in the practice area.

I wanted to do some research with psychiatric nurses and knew that my opportunity had come when I revisited the practice area. Research highlights, and provides a way of expressing, exploring and changing, all kinds of practice. I wanted psychiatric nursing to be highlighted to express itself and explore its practice. During my time as reliever, the regular weekly meetings I attended, along with the stories told in corridors or passing through the office, provided me with an opportunity to listen to the concerns expressed by experienced psychiatric nurses about their new role as DAOs.

It was through my conversations and contact with Annette Street, whom I had met in 1992 at the Wellington Polytechnic, that we came up with the idea of doing some research with the Hutt nurses on their role as DAOs. Annette is an experienced researcher and well known author in the nursing area but had not worked in the psychiatric field. I was just starting in the research area, but was well known in the psychiatric nursing area (in some places, anyway). So we decided we could be a good research team for this one.

The theme of the research

On 1 November 1992 the Mental Health (Compulsory Assessment and Treatment) Act became law in New Zealand and replaced the Mental Health Act 1969. The 1992 Act was passed with the purpose of legally redefining who could be detained and assessed because of their mental health status. The objective of the 1992 Act is clear in terms of:

(a) establishing the need for psychiatric treatment for a patient
(b) the most appropriate placement for that patient
(c) the rights of any persons subjected to compulsory assessment and treatment (O'Reagan 1992).

Under the Act a legally constituted role has been developed, that of the duly authorised officer (DAO). This position is generally carried out by psychiatric nurses, although other health professionals have been employed as DAOs. The duties of this DAO role have been articulated as being responsible to the director of area mental health services for the provision of:

• advice to the public concerning the operation of the Act and the services available for those suffering from mental disorder (section 37)
• practical advice in dealing with persons who may be mentally disordered (section 38)

- practical assistance with the assessment of proposed patients, and the care and treatment of patients on leave (section 39)
- assistance in taking or returning patients to their place of assessment or treatment (section 40) (O'Reagan 1992).

Community psychiatric nurses play a key role as duly authorised officers with changed roles and responsibilities giving them legal power to act in a way that is unique. They have become responsible for advice to the public, practical assessment of designated patients, care and treatment of patients on leave and assistance in taking or returning patients to their place of assessment or treatment.

As with all laws the development of the practices circumscribed by the law are detailed but subject to multiple legal and community interpretations. Nursing practices are multi-faceted, inconsistent and contingent, affected as much by custom and usage as by any legal or policy definition (Street 1990d, 1992). The Act has implications for the roles, responsibilities and practices of nurses who are appointed duly authorised officers because health planners and managers assume that, if the practices are described in legal and planning terms, the practitioners will be able to translate these criteria into appropriate expert practice. The assumption is based on an applied view of knowledge and reveals ignorance about the complexity of any nursing role and the inherent tensions and dilemmas in this context where a therapeutic, advocacy role has been broadened and legalised.

The pilot study investigation of the issues facing DAOs in the Hutt region provided evidence of the complexities and inconsistencies which are inherent in the Act and demonstrated the need for a more thorough investigation of the issues, and effects of the Act, on DAOs, on patients and on their families or care givers. As we learned that the department of mental health was collecting some statistical information on the use of DAOs in the community, we decided to explore various questions and problems inherent in the practice of the DAOs. This was a response to the concerns being discussed informally in any forums wherever DAOs gathered. Chris's experience had shown that there were many unexplored industrial, educational, policy, and legal issues with implications for practice. Chris and I formed a research team and clarified our research topic which became: 'Issues surrounding the practice of community mental health nurses using the Mental Health (Compulsory Assessment and Treatment) Act of 1992'.

Deciding on praxis research

To investigate the topic we needed to decide on the most appropriate method for the situation. We needed one that fitted the research question—a method which would enable us to uncover the issues contextually embedded in the practice of psychiatric nurses. We decided against a quantitative method such as a survey as we didn't understand the complexities of the new DAO role. We would not have been able to devise an appropriate questionnaire that would provide us with the information we wanted about how issues worked out for the nurses in the study.

For this project Chris and I decided that we needed an interactive, collaborative research method, a choice we were able to make because of our previous research experience and our understanding of the roles of clinical nurses and nursing practice. My experience of working with praxis research processes over the previous seven years had convinced me of the value of this form of research for clinical nurses intent on understanding and changing the dilemmas and inequities they encounter in their daily work (Street 1990b, 1991, 1992a, 1992b, 1992c, 1993). Nurses are performers whose work requires cognitive, psycho-social, technical, and physical skills along with the ability to co-ordinate the work of others. Nursing practice means that sophisticated clinical judgements are expressed through action and interaction. Nurses are also wonderful storytellers, and psychiatric nurses use stories and story analysis as part of their repertoire of practice skills. Chris and I were interested in a research design which valued the psychiatric nurse's skills of performance and storytelling.

We were also aware that a great many of the actions people perform are habitual and not the result of either conscious knowledge or choice. Some of these habitual actions can be reclaimed and restructured as a result of reflection, but some actions are caused by social conditions over which people have little control. When new legislation is introduced, new social conditions are created which cause changes in policies, procedures, roles and relationships along with changes in resource allocation and educational needs.

Praxis research endeavors to uncover both the systems of social relationships which determine the actions of individuals and the unanticipated consequences of these actions for the individual and society. Therefore praxis research was a useful method to examine the systems of social relationships for psychiatric nurses and their patients with the introduction of the Mental Health Act (Compulsory Assessment and Treatment) 1992.

The politics of the research performance

Praxis research methodologies regard the research act as a political act because it assumes that nurses are capable of reflecting upon the processes of their own nursing practice, in the light of power relationships, to uncover the ways they have unwittingly collaborated. The reflection requires not only an identification of the power games that other people play but a recognition of our own roles in the perpetuation of the oppressive practices of the status quo. It necessitates asking questions about our clinical, administrative, curriculum and research practices in order to identify how they produce dependence and perpetuate injustice and inequity. Reflection challenges us to move from perpetuating the hierarchical notions implicit in our 'us and them' mentalities to the development of the collective 'we', who care deeply about the provision of empowering, holistic health care. It requires people who are committed to 'making a difference'.

The pilot stage of the research was conducted using a PAR model which valued:

* reciprocity in research relationships
* negotiation of meaning
* theorising which spoke to the understandings and conditions of the mental health nurse participants.

The process was directed at identifying the complexity of practice issues which could be addressed in policy, social organisation and nursing practice. Praxis research is concerned with bridging the divide between theory and practice in such a way that the purpose of the researcher and the participants is not only to understand the world as it is experienced but, where appropriate, to improve it.

In this form of research the processes must always be under scrutiny like the topic. Praxis research demands that we critique what we are doing as we go along as a basis for improvement. There is a need for researchers and nurses to retreat from criticism of others as a strategy for dealing with difficulties, and join together positively in self-reflexive critique. As researchers, Chris and I kept not only field notes documenting the specific activities of the project but also journal notes which provided the basis for further reflection on our research practices.

For the pilot study we chose to use focus groups and semi-structured interviews. This choice enabled us to develop and critique stories of practice. We were then able to extrapolate the issues that came up in order to understand how they arose and interacted with each other in the complexity of clinical experience.

Assembling the research group

Praxis research does not use people as subjects of the research but involves the participants in the processes and analysis of the research. The pilot research strategy involved inviting the psychiatric nurses acting as DAOs in the Hutt region to take part in exploring their changed role. Initially Chris discussed our embryonic idea with Debbie Gell, a representative of the group of nurses we hoped would participate in the project. Debbie responded enthusiastically and agreed to speak about the project with the other members of the group. Her feedback was that the members were positive about the idea of participating in this form of research.

Gaining access

At this point we commenced the lengthy processes involved in getting a research project underway. As a team Chris and I were able to split the tasks. I was back working in Australia and so put my energy into designing a feasible short study which met our shared agendas. Meanwhile Chris approached the various regional administrators with a preliminary outline of the study to find out about ethical assessment and management permission. She recorded the process of then establishing the group like this:

On 2 June 1993 I met with the community mental health nurses as a group to discuss the proposed research project. The written outline I had drafted referred to the topic, the aim, the methodology and further issues to be addressed in relation to the development of the research. I had spoken to Debbie about the possibilities in regard to the topic of issues surrounding the practice of community mental health nurses using the new Mental Health Act, and she was enthusiastic about this. Annette and I had talked through ways we might collect data and so I included this in the draft outline. I had decided that it would provide a much tighter focus if each person had a draft document to work from initially, so that the time would be spent productively, as these nurses had a busy schedule and time was important to them. I also thought that it was important that they see that Annette and I had put some thought into this project already. (We were not mucking around here!)

The meeting went well and we discussed the topic and issues like consent, confidentiality, ownership of information and ethical considerations. Since two of the community mental health nurses were not present at this meeting the other group members agreed to consult with them and let me know the next week about whether or not the group was willing to participate in the project. I felt quite positive about the group and the way the meeting had gone.

The next week I heard all group members were willing to participate in the research. This was great news and I felt quite inspired. I organised an interview timetable and posted this out to Debbie who agreed to distribute it to the group members.

In this project Chris spoke with the nurses before formally approaching management because she was working with the nurses collaboratively to design the project. It was to be a participatory project and the focus and methods were developed interactively. Following on from this study we received funding to replicate it in other areas and to further develop the issues it had examined.

As the major study design was later approved by the funding body, the Health Research Council of New Zealand, we then managed the access process differently. After the feedback at the major conferences we were approached by various nursing managers of DAO services, to offer their services to participate in the larger study. Our further choice of areas was influenced by the need to include rural and cultural perspectives in our sample, so we were not able to accept all the offers. However it meant that we had contact people who managed local services and acted as sponsors to their organisation and to the senior manager.

In other circumstances I have written to the senior executive of an organisation who has then passed on the request to the appropriate person to set in motion the gate keeping processes. In one case the regional health director wanted to meet us and have an in depth discussion of the research design before it was handed on to the research co-ordinator for the region. There are no general rules about gaining access and it depends on the researcher's status as an insider or outsider to the organisation and also the relationships of sponsors and gatekeepers. The first rule is to do a reconnaissance and be flexible. Where research activities are new or different staff find themselves responsible for the research, it is important to recognise that expectations and processes can change rapidly. It is also valuable to remember to double check your information and the understanding you have of the process as it is possible to be given incorrect information. This can lead to confusion and stress and it may stop the research from proceeding. Chris recounts how the process of gate keeping and access worked for her in the first instance:

On 9 June I met with the manager of the service to seek support for the research. She hoped the service would benefit from the research and not just the community nurses and was happy for the nurses to use any information gained as long as management also had access to that information. We established that no client or staff names would be used. She also noted that the nurses would be talking about work done for the service and the clients so there was some discussion about responsibility and ownership.

We discussed ethical approval for the project and as this was a pilot project I understood she would seek out and gain ethical approval through local structures. The manager was very supportive of the project and of the idea that we might present some of the findings at the annual Psychiatric Nursing Conference to be held in Wellington in October.

The following week I met with the co-ordinator of the mental health nursing team to seek support and provide information. His concerns were similar to those of the manager and he too was supportive of the project. He did inquire as to whether there was any possibility of adding any other aspects to the research!

The only real 'hitch' was the ethical approval. When I had not heard back from the manager about ethical approval for the project I contacted her. It seems that I had misunderstood that she would get ethical approval for us! The approval that she had sought was from her manager for the project. This was disastrous news considering Annette was due to fly in from Australia in a week's time to start on the project and the interviews had been set up for the following week. It turned out that I had to get approval from the Wellington Ethics Committee and by all accounts this was not a five second procedure! Needless to say I set about this task with great gusto and immediately rang the secretary only to establish, via answer phone, that they only work there from Wednesday to Friday (this was Monday). By Wednesday every person I knew was aware that Chris was stressed out and was busy trying to get ethical approval for a project! Fortunately I went to see Owen Robinson, the then chairperson of the committee. He was most helpful and agreed to give the proposal prompt attention. I had done as much as I could by using the guidelines set out by the committee and having frantic discussions with Annette on the phone, email and fax (great phone bill at the end of the month—the hidden costs of research). The only other hitch was that the day I was trying to get managerial signatures was the day that the health system in New Zealand was turned on its head structurally and Regional Health Authorities and Crown Health Enterprises came into existence. Consequently there was some uncertainty as to who was managing at the time and whose signature would be valid!

As is evident from this account, Chris' first experience of managing the access processes was stressful. Since then she has managed much more complex situations with aplomb while being meticulous in following up every conversation. She confirms and double checks every appointment and procedure which we need to go through—an essential role in any research team.

Preliminaries and informed consent

When I arrived in New Zealand from Australia, Chris and I met with the participants in a preliminary focus group meeting which identified the broad issues to be developed further in the interviews, reiterated the ethical issues and obtained informed consent. Although the group members had been given a copy of the research protocol and participant's consent form we had not asked them to sign their consent until they had met with us. This allowed the participants an opportunity to re-shape the research design to better meet their interests and needs as participants. The delay in signing the consent form also provided a cooling off period so that participants could think through the implications of their participation in the research. No documentation of individual contributions was collected until after the consent forms were signed, although the issues which the group members raised and wished to address within the research were noted as were their schedules and times of availability for interview and subsequent groups.

Gendered responses

There were four men and four women participating in the study. The women were all more experienced as psychiatric nurses and in the community role. It was interesting to see how gender made a difference in how information was provided during the study. The focus groups were dominated by the male participants and more discussion time was spent on topics of greater interest to them, such as financial reimbursement. However the interviews with the women were much more comprehensive and took much longer than with the men. The women tended to be more reflective which may have been indicative of their greater experience. However they rarely challenged the views espoused by the men during the focus groups even though some of the opinions they provided during the interviews would have suggested that their ideas differed. As researchers we dealt with this during subsequent focus groups by raising the matters again and by providing a variety of quotes which provided complementary and conflicting views on them. The openly ideological nature of praxis inquiry means that not only socially constituted nursing hierarchies need to be examined but the hierarchies of the research process itself. Researchers claiming an intention to improve a given situation need to be careful that they are not perpetuating the oppression of the research participants by disempowering them in the research process. Exalting the theoretical constructions of the researcher over the values and understandings held by practitioners endorses the gap between theory and practice. However it is also important that the participants' views are challenged when the researchers find discrepancies between the evidence they are working with and the participant's view of the situation. During the analysis of the interview transcripts, it became evident that gender was an issue for the female nurses, for the patients and for Chris and I during our work with the focus groups. However when we raised it with the group, the men strongly argued that it was not an issue and the women did not challenge them. We were prepared to accept that they did not consider gender an issue in relation to the DAO role but we also wanted to reflect our own analysis in the reporting. So we reported that although gender was not considered an issue by the participants we held a different view and would explore this dimension further in a larger study.

The research script

The introductory meeting was followed by an individual semi-structured interview with each participant. These interviews lasted for at least an hour and provided the opportunity for community psychiatric nurses to articulate their experiences prior and subsequent to, the enactment of the Mental Health Act 1992.

There was no fixed wording or sequencing of the interview questions, however an interview schedule was developed to enable us to collect information on the same areas from each nurse. The semi-structured interview schedule included questions from the following categories:

- Background demographics
  Some background information was collected to help the researchers understand how the DAOs' prior education and experience informed their comments.
- Knowledge questions
  The DAOs were asked questions to elicit what factual knowledge the nurses had regarding the Mental Health Act and their role in particular.
- Narrative questions
  The researchers asked the participants to contextualise their comments by providing stories which explained the issues from their personal experience. This enabled the researchers and participants to explore the social structures and relationships inherent in the issues under consideration.
- Contrast questions
  The participants were asked to provide stories which demonstrated the comparisons between their experiences under the 1969 and 1992 Mental Health Acts.
- Opinion and value questions
  Questions were designed to understand the cognitive and interpretive processes which participants and researchers were using.
- Challenge questions
  The research participants were also asked questions which were designed to elicit the taken for granted assumptions underlying their responses, and provide opportunities to challenge or respond to interpretations as they emerged.

As our focus was on isolating significant issues the nurses were able to work with us and with each other to identify issues and articulate how they functioned. The storytelling process provided us all with the opportunity to reflect on our own experiences in a supportive environment and think about why things happened in the way that they did, what our roles were in continuing the situation and what actions could be taken to improve it. The process enabled the nurse participants to have their experiences validated and offered them an opportunity to consider how their practices might be reconstructed. The participants gave graphic examples of the complexities of their work. For example, one DAO described how under-resourcing can put nurses and others in the community at risk of physical danger.

I'm running around. I haven't got a cell phone, I mean that's one of the issues [lack of resources]. One situation when the police were there the woman was locked in the house. The curtains were drawn. We didn't know whether she was self-harming—reports were that she had put a pair of scissors in her mouth and was bleeding from the mouth, etc., and I was running up and down from this neighbour's house—who let me use the phone—it was 200 yards away—trying to get the GP, negotiate with the hospital and the consultant psychiatrist. This is on a Sunday 'cos she was doing her garden and said, 'Can't it wait till tomorrow?'...You are running around like a bloody idiot and the police are looking at you thinking, 'Christ what a set up he works for!' You're asking too much of one person to do the forms, co-ordinate, it's too much really. [It's] a bit like a taxi service and the messenger in this Act.

Stories such as these which contextualised the issues were not only collected, but the participants were invited to identify what the issues were for them.

The process of analysis

Praxis or participatory action researchers are concerned that the theory developed through the process not only deconstruct the world but reconstruct it (Stanley 1990). Lather (1991:55) argues that theory 'adequate to the task of changing the world must be open ended, non-dogmatic, speaking to, and grounded in, the circumstances of everyday life'. It must be developed reciprocally and the findings need to be disseminated in such a form that the research participants, and others in their place, can understand and use them. In this way the findings are directed at those people involved in the situation—whether in nursing, management or policy—rather than at the research community.

The material was analysed not only for what was included in the transcripts but also for material relevant to the Act that was excluded, omitted or ignored in the interviews with the nurses. During the analysis Chris and I identified each issue as it occurred in the data. We organised the issues into major groupings and identified the relationships between them. After the first round we had a list of major issues with many subordinate issues grouped with them. The major groupings looked like this:

- definitional problems in the Act
- lack of cultural safety
- co-ordination difficulties with mental health and community service providers
- medical dominance affecting the assessment process
- physical danger to DAOs
- strain on care givers and other community resources
- lack of initial orientation and continuing education
- inadequate resources for the service
- gendered constructions of mental health affecting the treatment of women
- the role in isolated rural communities
- the lack of appropriate remuneration for the additional DAO role

We reviewed the transcripts and found further evidence of the different dimensions of these issues. Then we located specific stories or comments which appeared to place the issues in context.

The interviews were followed by a focus group discussion of an hour. This provided the participants with the opportunity to hear the researchers' feedback on the analysis to date and make further comments and contributions. The feedback was given in the form of an explanation of each issue, the major points which had emerged and the key quotes which might be used to illustrate the issue further. The process of feedback was very interactive as the research participants corrected and extended Chris and my knowledge of the situation. These further comments were analysed and became part of the draft report. The draft report was written to show what we had found and our analysis of the key issues. For example, the area of training was an area which the DAOs were very vocal about. They stated that they had inadequate orientation or training and this was of particular concern with the need to be conversant with the processes of judicial hearings—a new and frightening experience for most nurses. We reported their comments as:

The DAOs were clear about what kind of training would be valuable. They felt that those training days where they sat and listened to experts were not very useful as they usually covered the material which the expert thought was necessary but this rarely coincided with what those in practice saw as the main concerns.

One area of concern was the judicial reviews introduced under the new Mental Health Act. The members of the Hutt group discussed this during a focus group and raised the following concerns:

- That they were often made to feel as if they were guilty because of the adversarial nature of the review.

- That they were unaware of court procedures and the proper forms of address.
- That they learn how to write court reports and to understand the requirements of writing for legal purposes.
- That the workshops be generated from the issues which the DAOs dealt with rather than what lawyers and others needed to deal with under the Act.
- That the workshops be experiential (Street 1993:11).

A further focus group validated the data from this draft report to be used in the report at two conferences. A workshop conducted at the National Psychiatric Nursing Conference enabled the issues located in the Hutt region to be explored, challenged, critiqued and confirmed by DAOs from all over New Zealand. A series of recommendations were developed for further discussion, and subsequent adoption with minimal modifications, at the DAO conference 'Through the Looking Glass'.

The critical review

Writing from a critical perspective Brian Fay (1977) contends that it is not only important for people to come to a new self-understanding as the basis for altering social arrangements, but also that the manner in which they come to adopt this new 'guiding idea' is important. Processes of collaborative dialogue are identified as the most desirable basis. According to Fay the conditions by which the groups of people who experience themselves as oppressed by race, gender, sexism, or ageism make a change in their basic self-conception is through:

> an environment of trust, openness, and support in which one's own perceptions and feelings can be made properly conscious to oneself, in which one can think through one's experiences in terms of a radically new vocabulary which expresses a fundamentally different conceptualisation of the world, in which one can see the particular and concrete ways that one unwittingly collaborates in producing one's own misery, and in which one can gain the emotional strength to accept and act on one's new insights (Fay 1977:232).

Here Fay is alerting us to the kind of collaborative group climate by which individuals can become self-aware and begin to engage in critique. He reminds us that this process requires us to re-examine our language, and the myths and concepts which our words represent, and then develop new language to describe our new understandings with. He challenges us to recognise the ways in which we co-operate with others to maintain and daily re-create the situations which we experience as injustice. And, finally, Fay emphasises the process of gaining emotional strength in order that we may both accept and act upon our new insights.

The nurses who participated in the focus group were both interested and amazed that others had the same experiences and views. Although they regularly met together for administrative matters they did not meet to discuss the stories and implications of their practice. The research process alerted group members to the strength they had as a group, and although this was a short project some of the issues were then addressed further by the group through negotiation and industrial action. The group members were also clearer on the issues as a result of participating in the research. They were then able to provide some direction for other DAOs who had experienced the same difficulties but had not had any systematic way of investigating them.

Lather (1985:8) reminds us 'that we are both shaped by and shapers of our world'. She argues that we need research designs that:

> allow us to reflect on how our value commitments insert themselves into our empirical work. Our own frameworks of understanding need to be critically examined as we look for the tensions and contradictions they might entail...the search is for theory which grows out of context embedded data, not in a way that rejects a prior theory, but in a way that keeps it from distorting the logic of evidence. Theory is too often used to protect us from the awesome complexity of the world (Lather 1985:25).

Reflective and participatory processes are demanding of researchers as they require an examination of the complex realities of practice as they are known. This kind of critique does not contain well recognised problems waiting to be solved. Instead it poses dilemmas with equally acceptable solutions, which is consistent with different value stances and ways of understanding the world of clinical practice. Reflection does not begin with a search for answers but with a search for questions (Freire 1972). In this instance many questions were raised concerning the DAO role, the industrial conditions, the definitional problems of the Mental Health Act and the effect on the therapeutic and advocacy role previously a feature of the role of the community psychiatric nurse. Questions were also raised concerning the conduct of the research.

Although we talked about being collaborative and reciprocal, the success of the pilot study resided more in the timely nature of the question, the method of investigation and the opportunity to validate the findings nationally. The study provided the group members with information, a communication process, and the opportunity to use the findings of the research in industrial action at a time when they had grave concerns and a desire to act on them. The research participants were all proud of their contribution to the research and agreed that the findings reflected their concerns and their experiences of the issues. They were very keen to be named on the front of the report in recognition of their involvement. They also found that the research was 'good fun' and 'we should do more of that'.

Although the study was firmly under the control of the researchers, the wider dissemination of the findings through the interactive workshops, contributed further to the understanding and validation of the preliminary findings and provided some direction for other DAOs in New Zealand. This wider validation process meant that the research was authenticated in other quarters and because of its timely nature it has since influenced legal, industrial and educational initiatives, receiving attention from key policy makers.

The collaborative aspect of the research was in the development, analysis and validation of the data with the participating DAOs. The reciprocity was in the process of negotiating the meanings of the data with the Hutt nurses, with the wider DAO community and with policy makers, managers and educators. The further research funding has involved us with a new set of research problems to negotiate—new access processes, different ethical expectations, contrasting structures, specific rural and cultural issues to be worked through. We have reflected on our changed roles as researchers and the processes we initiate and structure, and this is an ongoing reflexive process.

8. Journalling

But why do I have to write about my nursing practice? This question is one of the first I encounter when I ask nurses to write what I call 'descriptive accounts' of their nursing practice. A simple answer to the question is that in the act of writing we can record all our thoughts, feelings and actions for ourselves and others. The record is then available for analysis, and to provide a picture of our personal and professional development in relation to an issue of concern. In effect this is an argument for the collection of research data on ourselves as professional people and into the socio-cultural practice worlds which we inhabit.

The first hurdle is the fact that writing for research in this way is often an unfamiliar activity for clinical nurses. As with any venture into a new area the proposal that nurses write short accounts generally elicits some anxiety and apprehension. When individuals understand that this anxiety is shared by their colleagues, and that writing clear descriptive accounts is a skill that we as mentors can teach them, they are free to begin to work with us.

Beginning to write

A common difficulty expressed by nurses is the problem of arranging writing time in busy schedules. As one nurse reported:

I went to the shop and bought a book before I came on the afternoon shift. I was determined to start writing some descriptive accounts. At 5.30 p.m. I decided to sit down and write about the incident which had happened earlier in the afternoon. I wrote two sentences, got interrupted, came back, wrote three more lines and then had to go off again. I didn't do any more for two days. Then I wrote a few more lines but it is pretty pathetic [hands book to me] so I thought maybe you could help me.

It is evident that the difficulty of beginning to write is not only related to the effort required to set aside time to write, but also to the sneaky suspicion, which many of us hold, that the effort may not be worthwhile. In our world of electronic communication, for many adults, letter writing is being replaced by telephones, tape recorders, videos, or fax machines. Work roles have been re-structured so that few occupations require sustained descriptive and analytical writing. When confronted with the need to engage in descriptive writing, it is not surprising that many people secretly doubt their capacity to do it. Adults such as nurses, whose occupations demand concise and carefully constructed reporting procedures, may doubt the relevance of an outpouring of words. Others have reported a concern that 'it is self-centered' to write about their own professional practice. However, for those who are prepared to take the risk and face themselves on paper, descriptive accounts can form the basis of research into the self as a professional person in a socially constructed work setting, and provide the necessary data to facilitate systematic and rational change.

Taking the risk to describe our practice on paper is not easy to do as our internal censors often interfere with our presentation of self in a written account. Initially we can find ourselves writing in the truncated shorthand form in which we think about that particular habitual practice. We may find that we begin with explanations or justifications as we carry on an internal dialogue. It is often the presence of the internal censor at work, in the writing of the account, which can prompt the novice account writer to look back over what is written and think 'so what?' The challenge is to provide enough detailed description of practice to stand back and critically examine them as if they were an account of the actions of someone else. Support during this introductory phase is often found through the development of collaborative relationships, which enable nurses to share their accounts with another more experienced person acting as a guide in the process. As one nurse recounts:

Over the last few days I have come home, sat down and written about my work. It read clearly to me, although I wasn't getting much out of the process. Today I swapped journals with my friend who has been doing journalling as part of an education course. She astounded me by saying she didn't really understand what I had written. I re-read what I had written and realised that each day I had been planning what I would write as I drove home. By the time I arrived I had already worked out how to get the details down with the least amount of effort.

This afternoon I sat down and re-wrote the accounts out in detail in the way that my friend had been doing in her journal. I began to enjoy the process. It really made me think. Already I can see things in what I have written that I hadn't expected or known about myself as a nurse.

There are a number of issues that are obvious and I feel that there are more if I look carefully.

It is clear that the capacity to describe an engagement in professional practice comprehensively is an essential part of developing researchable data. One nurse who has been engaged in participatory research says:

Yes, because as nurses, I mean, that's one of the things. I did this lecture on our research, and one of the things I said was how as nurses we're used to being verbal, we start doing hand over, we're not good at writing nursing notes particularly. We're not good at writing, and I found that my accounts had improved over time. Now I look back and I shudder at them [the early attempts] because we're not taught anything to do with writing research accounts. I mean the words that we use!

When working with nurses who have found it difficult to uncover all the taken for granted aspects of their clinical practice because of insufficient descriptive data, I have found it useful to work with a series of basic questions which expand their perceptions of other aspects of encounters with patients. The questions generally covered the following aspects:

- Setting—Where was I? What could I see, smell, hear and feel in the setting?
- Personnel—Who was I involved with? Who else was in range of the interaction?
- Content of the activity—What was I doing? Why?
- Account of the interaction—What did I do or say first? What happened next? How did it happen? What was said by whom to whom? What responses were elicited?
- What was I thinking and feeling at the time?

Focusing on these questions developed new habits of description which replace the established habits of mental shorthand. When I have the opportunity I ask nurses to sit with their eyes closed and relive a particular experience in their imagination. I use the questions listed above as the basis for the exercise. I then ask the nurses to tell us their stories orally and we ask questions for clarification. Then I ask them to write down the stories they have just told. In this way the story is fresh and some of the taken for granted assumptions have been identified during the discussion.

With other groups I may begin by asking nurses to recount stories on tape for transcription. I ask questions which help the nurses elaborate assumptions and missing detail and then hand them back the reconstructed accounts as a preliminary exercise to demonstrate the rich material in the accounts. As nurses develop experience with descriptive material as a source of research data they may decide to move on to the practice of keeping a personal and professional journal.

Journals are generally private documents which contain material that can be shared with sympathetic colleagues or critical friends. They enable the writers to collect the history of their own practice over time, a record of actions, thoughts, insights, ideas, quotes, issues and the cathartic material generated through the recording of feelings. Journals can provide a source of research data into the professional life of the writers, into the socio-cultural situation in which the work is practised and into the social relationships which pervade the context (Holly 1987). I intend to write about journal writing in detail to demonstrate the manner by which journals can be structured as research.

A question of style

Historically much of the education in nursing practice has been taught on the assumption that there is a correct way to carry out an activity. When nurses bring this history to the activity of keeping a journal then they are often concerned with questions regarding the right way to write their journals. Observation of many journals has confirmed in me the conviction that no two journals are alike, in the same way as no two people are alike. It is through the process of freeing ourselves to express ourselves in our own unique ways that we can develop records that will enable us to research ourselves and our practices. This freedom means different things for different people. For one woman a process of bombarding her page with different words written at different angles and of different sizes helps her unlock her unconscious and examine previously censored values, ideas and theories. A number of people find it useful to use a large double spread book and write their descriptions in one column and their commentary or analysis in another. Some people break this up still further with sections for bright ideas, proposed actions, quotes from reading or the identification of issues. Some journals look neat, others appear messy with arrows and writing everywhere. Some contain pictures and photos, some contain illustrations or idiosyncratic diagrams, while other people use colored inks, highlighting pens and margin notes. If the content is intended to reflect the uniqueness of the individual as a professional person, then surely that format and style should also be representative of that person.

An important element of journal writing is the acknowledgment that the process of writing makes conscious the unconscious within us. For some people this may take months to draw out. Professional practice necessitates language which fits within specified conventions of brevity, accuracy, uniformity and structured formats. These professional writing activities are generally produced for a wider audience than just ourselves and so we generally activate our internal censors to inhibit creative and private forms of recording and reporting. This censoring is appropriate for these professional activities but it appears that many of us have learnt the censoring process too well. When we have the freedom to express ourselves, many of us act as if someone is looking over our shoulder to examine our neatness or precision. After six months of regular journal keeping some of the professionals I have worked with reported difficulties in allowing themselves the luxury of free and sincere expression of their feelings, attitudes and values. In contrast, others took control of their journals from the first day and filled them with their writings about themselves and their work. I find it interesting that a common claim among people who have examined and expressed themselves freely in their journals is that they regard their journal as their friend. This friendship represents the satisfaction which develops through knowing oneself more fully, both personally and professionally, and through a growing acknowledgment of the silent and unconscious parts which have been previously ignored.

Freezing the action

The act of writing about practice enables the writer to freeze the action. Action which is frozen in a journal can be examined from all aspects, particularly those which are on the fringes of consciousness. When Kate, an intensive care unit nurse, had to have her own son admitted to ICU she wrote in her journal:

Sean required another dose of adrenalin, however he deteriorated soon after. It was then that the doctor mentioned the 'T' word. 'if he deteriorates again Kate, we'll have to tube him'. The lump in my throat grew larger and the tears began to fall down my cheeks. All I could see before me was difficult intubation, an empty oxygen cylinder, prolonged intubation time, subglottic stenosis—the list went on. Sure enough Sean's air entry was reducing, he was more lethargic and starting to become clammy. A tube was now imminent. However, a child had deteriorated in the next room and as the doctor was unable to be in two places at one time, another dose of racemic adrenalin was essential for Sean. The fight against the mask was now minimal and my baby was frighteningly pale. My whole world now felt so fragile. I was experiencing what so many parents had felt before me and, as an ICU nurse, I had never realised the gravity of these feelings. This was my baby and I felt powerless to help him. I couldn't hold back the tears any longer and reached for the shoulder of Sean's nurse, my colleague...Miraculously, Sean settled into a deep sleep and his breathing became less and less labored. This last dose of racemic adrenalin had pushed him in the right direction and now the image of the dreaded tube was starting to fade. The weight on my shoulders eased. I looked around the room at the parents of these desperately ill children—how in the hell did they cope for days on end, often with little hope?

By bringing into the foreground of her consciousness, those things which she had previously left unexamined, how it really felt for the parents of seriously ill babies admitted to ICU, Kate froze the action and became aware of an important insight which was to change her nursing practice. The act of writing itself helped Kate to order her thinking and acknowledge the insight more fully.

It is impossible for anyone to write about the totality of the experience. Writing about professional practice is always a process of making choices among multiplicities. A common complaint from novice journal-keepers is:

Writing is frustrating. I really can't tell the whole story. I leave out so much.

Since writing journal accounts involves choices, it enables us to record things which are significant to us and ignore parts of our daily existence that we don't want to record or attend to. It is important to recognise that as reflection is action oriented it would be impossible and unnecessary to confront all the chaos of our personal and professional lives at one time. Therefore keeping a journal allows us to choose the focus on our practice and examine it thoroughly. The examination may mean that we may think of an incident as a complex photo. We may choose to enlarge different parts of the photo and shift the focus from one to another. We may decide to blur some parts and examine the detail in others. We can move from the whole to the parts and back again. It is in this process of re-focusing that we can discover unknown or unconscious elements which contribute to a clearer picture.

Locating the autopilot and the taken for granted assumptions

As we write freely and descriptively about ourselves and our work, we can uncover the 'autopilot' which guides much of our day. The autopilot can unlock our stream of consciousness, the one-way running conversation most of us conduct in our heads all day, everyday. One nurse described the discovery of her autopilot like this:

I was tired after work and, as I was new to journalling and didn't want to forget to do it, I sat down and quickly wrote an account of some of my shift. My husband came in and asked what I was doing so I showed it to him. He gave it back and told me that he couldn't understand it anyway. I felt stunned as I hadn't written any nursing jargon. I asked him to tell me what he meant. He picked it up and read through it making comments like 'What does that mean? What is the connection between this and that? Why did you do this?' As I started to explain things to him I became aware of the fact that much of what I had written didn't make sense because I had written as I had acted—on autopilot. I hadn't censored it but I had skipped over important details. I sat down after tea and wrote it all up again descriptively so that my husband could understand it. As we read it through I was totally amazed at the things that jumped out at me. It really hit me then how a good descriptive account could enable you to do research on yourself. Up till then I hadn't really believed that I could do it.

The discovery of the autopilot leads to the recognition of the taken for granted assumptions implicit in our understandings of our socio-cultural world. Andrew recorded an experience in his journal which revealed that he held a taken for granted assumption that the only effective way for a group to function was if members stuck to an agenda. He was attending a self-help group for the first time as a participant but was known to some members in his professional capacity as a nurse. After writing a full description of the meeting he reflected:

During the entire discussion I found difficulty with letting the conversation flow from topic to topic, without bringing it back to the point. If often made me nervous and tense as I couldn't stand the unstructured nature of it all. I guess I like to be in control, and when I see an agenda I want to pursue it. (Of course this is what I did on the ward, pursue my agenda, which to a certain extent created a situation of dependency)...In the end [at the meeting] I was quite amazed at some of the solutions or plans they came up with, which were what I would have suggested anyway. The central ideas were theirs. The time scale was theirs.

Writing about the experience of attending the self-help group enabled Andrew to identify and clarify the taken for granted assumptions which he had unconsciously endorsed in his expectations of functional groups. He was also able to transfer his understanding of the implications of these assumptions to his habitual practices in his work setting. He was able to recognise that his need to take control of proceedings created a situation where others depended on him to do their thinking for them. By examining what the group had achieved without his control, he was able to recognise that his assumption was invalid and that other processes could bring about a similar result without creating dependency.

An engagement in this kind of indepth search for meanings can reveal the habitual actions, patterns, contradictions and regularities within our daily routinised work. These things become apparent when we take the time to write and think about what we do, particularly under pressure of time. Andrew recorded this in his journal after a discussion with Jenny, an RN, about the previous shift when we had been conducting a participant observation session with her:

Jenny approached me today to discuss last Wednesday when she worked with Annette and I on the ward. She said that she found it very stressful to sit with us and discuss the issues related to the management of the disabled child. When we discussed this issue she said that she did not have trouble sitting down and spending time with us talking, but felt very guilty that the other nurses were picking up her work. She said that prior to our arrival on the ward she had told the nurses in sections 3 and 4 that we were coming to the ward and that she would be spending time with us. When I asked her how they had responded to this plan she said that they were not at all negative about the prospect of her absence during the morning, but I sensed from her that she did not really feel that they were overwhelming in their support. When you think about it, what would you say anyway? 'No you can't'. Nurses don't often like to be openly confrontational with each other....Sally said that as soon as Jenny started work she went as hard as she could to get as much as she could 'finished'. To me it was evident that despite assurances of support Jenny either had to complete most if not all of her own work, either because she was not confident in the support of her colleagues and feared the consequent violence, or because she has an implicit difficulty with being involved in activities, like those which Annette and I wish to pursue, when there are tasks relating to patient care awaiting completion. I think both options have some currency in the situation.

When we talked about Jenny's experience of analysing her work as a nurse, she acknowledged that it had been limited in the extreme. The only time she spent any time on duty discussing her work, or even reading about the various conditions suffered by the children in her care, was when it was so quiet on the ward that the other available options were reading *New Idea* or watching TV. In reality what this means is that involvement in taking time to develop your knowledge/understanding is not highly valued by Jenny, especially when compared to completing the important tasks/rituals associated with what nurses call 'patient care'. In this respect Jenny's values reflect the values of the wider nursing culture which values doing above thinking or reflecting or analysing [certainly as a nurse I can identify with this having my own history of being a well meaning but rampant 'activist'].

Here Andrew was reflecting on the clash between the research culture and task centered clinical nursing. Researchers value opportunities to investigate before they commence action. This causes distress to nurses who inhabit a world where the unexpected problem means they strive to keep up with an imaginary timetable of activities. The attitude is reflected in language such as 'I'm ahead today'. By recording the instance in his journal Andrew was not only able to unpick the situation as it was for Jenny, but also the effect of nursing culture on how Jenny and her colleagues prioritised their work. Andrew was able to see how he had changed and how he was now able to analyse nursing culture from the perspective of a researcher rather than someone providing patient care. It gave an insight into the taken for granted assumptions underpinning the two cultures.

Another nurse, engaged in researching collaborative action with an established community group, demonstrates the way in which an examination of her attitudes and actions in her journal helps her confront the contradictions inherent in them. She writes:

I found tonight I was back to my old role of trying to direct the group. I felt frustrated. I did not feel we were achieving something really concrete. Yet in a way, by Sarah venting her frustration and anger, the meeting brought up the hidden agendas of the group which have never been openly discussed before. When Joy suggested the group meet without me I felt quite taken aback. Almost like, 'How dare they'. I think it was because Joy said that she thought the 'group members' only should meet. I was under the illusion/hope that I too was a group member. So I wanted to be the separate superior professional, and one of the gang. Some contradiction!

This woman was recognising the difficulties of adjusting to her role as researcher in the group, and the implications of her attitudes and actions upon the role. Her journal became invaluable as she examined the hidden meanings behind her own actions and reactions. In the process of writing comprehensively, dilemmas and contradictions surface which illuminate the sociocultural world in which we live and work.

However facing ourselves on paper is sometimes a painful process and requires the support of others, particularly someone experienced to help us move beyond the habitual, and what it means to us, to a place where we can initiate permanent change. As one nurse reflected:

And our research involved journalling, and reflecting on our practices as nurses looking after children who sustain burn injuries. [We looked at] the procedures we performed on them, and subsequent pain and discomfort and anxiety that we caused them due to our nursing practices. And by journalling those, we looked at those objectively, with a lot of backup from our researcher, who really worked us through all that stuff, all those issues...At the time we just didn't see clearly...we were still stuck in, 'Well this is how it's done, how we've done it', and to really start criticising your own practices really means that you were criticising part of yourself, because you'd allowed it to happen. That was a really hard process for us, but the researcher really supported us in that, and basically the research came up with all these really good strategies to overcome some of the problems. We've changed procedures, and it also changed the people in the groups' attitude about pain, and its effective management.

Telling the story

Keeping a journal is a means of telling the story of professional practice over time. An examination of any personal or professional journal will reveal not only the actions, feelings and rationales of the writer, but will include valuable information about the context, the politics and other people who in any way impact on the professional life of the journal keeper. Narrative journal accounts are crafted in ways which lend themselves to multi-dimensional analysis. The language appropriated by the journal keeper is governed by social and ideological processes.

We use language which contains meaning for us and which reflects our socially constructed forms of thinking and acting. The culture of nursing has constructed different forms of thinking and acting. Language use reflects the professional cultural meanings. Nurses have an intimate involvement with the bodies of their patients, and this is evident in the vocabulary they use to describe their patients, themselves, and the situation. Nursing accounts abound in adjectives which describe the observable physical appearance of the patient, which has rich meaning for themselves and for other nurses. However accounts often develop a bio-psycho-social slant which neglects the cultural and intellectual aspect of their patients.

These kinds of culturally derived meanings can determine the ways in which nurses think about their professional roles. As the nursing role has expanded and changed, nurses are left grappling with new ways of describing themselves. As they examine their language they can identify ways in which the traditions of the past linger in the unconscious of the present. According to one nurse:

This woman had been described as a difficult patient and so I was apprehensive when I went into her room. I asked her how she was and she burst into tears. When I asked her what the matter was she just slumped into her bed facing toward the wall. Her face was very red and I noticed that she had clenched her fists. Another nurse came by and said, 'That's what she is like all the time. Won't tell you anything. And always rude and demanding.' I went over and sat by her bed and told her how sorry I was to see her so unhappy and that, although I couldn't wave a magic wand to change things, I would like to hear what she had to say so that we could work together to help her. After a time she began to stutter at me. Then she gave up trying to speak. Although I had other things to do I decided to just sit with her. After she calmed down she began to speak slowly. It was apparent that she had a bad stammer and it took time to let her say what she wanted to. She didn't understand what the doctors were doing to her and she was afraid that she would die. After I explained her condition and the treatment regime she began to relax. I told her that although her condition was serious it was not life threatening. Her color had improved so I sat her up comfortably so she could see the TV. She thanked me over and over for listening to her and explained that when she was anxious she could barely talk without stammering, but that she had disguised it by giving orders which didn't need much explanation. When I think about it I really didn't do anything much. I mean I was only talking to her, not working.

This is a typical story of a transformative nursing encounter. The changed perceptions of the nursing role has meant that nurses are being encouraged to spend time communicating with their patients instead of concentrating on those physical tasks which need to be done for the patient. However, two sentences ('Although I had other things to do I decided to just sit with her' and 'I mean I was only talking to her, not working') illuminate some of the symbolic content apparent in her story. This nurse strongly supports the need to spend time communicating yet written down, her language usage reveals an unconscious adherence to the belief that communicating with patients is not work. This account also demonstrates the use of multiple voices. As we read the account, we are taken into the thoughts and actions of the nurse, the patient, and a nursing colleague. We are presented with a first person, verbatim account of the comment by the nursing colleague and a summarised account of the interactive communication between nurse and patient. This record displays not only the speech but also the actions ('She just slumped into her bed facing toward the wall'; 'She gave up trying to speak'). It also reveals rationales and judgements made by nurse and patient:

It was apparent that she had a bad stammer and it took time to let her say what she wanted to. She didn't understand what the doctors were doing to her and she was afraid that she would die. After I explained her condition and the treatment regime she began to relax.

The narrative enables readers to place themselves in the story and understand and analyse it from the evidence presented like a novel. As a journal develops, stories appear which unfold similar themes even if the content of the story appears quite different. Stories which contain dialogue verbatim can often reveal values in use which contradict or depart from the individual's espoused values. As a researcher working with groups of nurses, I espouse the value of negotiated decision making and yet as I wrote about working with a new group I found myself revisiting old patterns of controlling behavior:

Well I blew it again today. I was tired and frustrated even before the group began. They insist on meeting at such an inconvenient time for me. These shifts drive me mad. Susie started to apologise for not having set up the practice interviews with her colleagues. As she was the one who had insisted on managing these interviews, I was not too impressed, but instead of working to find out what the real reason was I went for her:

Susie: Sorry Annette, I didn't have time to do what I said I'd do.

Annette: (thinks, 'She had 3 weeks!'). Well how will we manage without that information?

Susie: Well I don't think it is a good idea anyway.

Annette: But it was your idea.

Susie (defensively): Yes but I thought about it after, and I think we should do a survey.

Annette (coolly): I wasn't aware that you knew how to plan and conduct a survey.

Susie: I can't, but you can show us today.

Annette: I thought we had all agreed that a survey is inappropriate for this research question, as we don't know enough about the situation to even begin to plan some decent questions, and we don't have enough skill to do a proper analysis. Or was I mistaken?

Susie: Yes but I didn't do mine because I was on nights.

Annette: Well Susie I am just not prepared to put all the effort into teaching you how to do a survey when it won't get you the information that you need. Now what I think we should do is this...

And then with the knowledge that I had been inappropriate I went on to explain again the procedure for the 'conversation with a purpose' style interviews and then demonstrated a practice interview with another nurse. The group responded well and all had a practice at doing an interview on tape with each other before we finished. Last session I had worked hard with the group outlining all the data collection strategies, and Susie had pushed to launch into some preliminary interviews. This time, instead of getting Susie to talk further about why she had changed her mind and favoured a survey, I just pushed her into the data collection strategy that I deemed most valuable. I took control with my researcher's power, and it wasn't until Marj admitted that she had supported Susie's view of the survey because it felt safer, and she didn't have the confidence to do the interviews that I really understood what was happening. When I demonstrated the interview process, and then gave them all a chance to practise in the group, the atmosphere changed, and at the end they went off very enthusiastically with their tape to listen to. I could have managed that better and been more consistent with my espoused value of negotiation. If I had let Susie and the others air their ideas more, I would have heard their concerns and not had to work so hard to get on track again.

Reflection upon this kind of data enables the journal keeper to begin to comprehend the complexity of the intersubjective meanings hidden within the account of interaction. It is this telling the story and then systematically reflecting upon yourself in action in the narrative that constitutes the process of distancing. Different people develop different strategies to manage this distancing. Some begin each journal entry with a salutation or end with a signing off. When one nurse was asked the reason why she always signed her name at the end of each account, she responded:

That's an interesting question. I don't know why really—I just did it the first time and I have kept going…I guess if I am honest I think of my journal as representing 'me' to me. I guess that is the objectifying process which we have discussed. When I start writing I just let go and get as much off my chest as I can. After that first bit I guess I start to step back and talk to myself. I guess that's why I never start with anything like 'Dear Journal' but I always end by signing my name. At the end I am looking in on myself and my work.

It is through a process of analysis and reflection of these viewpoints that the individual is able to locate his or her own perspective and the meanings ascribed to it. Journalling as a dialogue between the objective and subjective self is a common practice.

Identifying and owning practices, values and feelings

Journalling is a process which enables us to engage in the process of listening to, owning and assessing values and feelings. This valuing and ownership can often occur as we learn to identify the ways we have repressed our values and feelings in the face of others' expectations. Writing about her experiences in hospital, one new mother was able to identify that she felt anxious about taking her baby home because he had been ill and she felt unsure of managing any recurrence of symptoms.

Now that everything looks OK, I'm glad, but a bit worried in case I don't know what to do if he gets any symptoms back again at home, but I guess there will be a chance to ask, before we are bundled out into the big wide world again.

As result of writing this, this mother was able to prepare herself for discharge teaching by planning what questions she wanted answers to. It enabled her to take charge and to feel more in control of the situation for herself and her new baby.

Reclaiming the historical self

This is the culmination of a narrative of present practices and the historical formation of these present practices and comes about as the result of dialogue with yourself. The narrative process of telling your own history, the history of the key actors in your story, and the historical development of the context is essential in disclosing your unspoken knowledge to yourself.

Journal keepers often begin with a potted history of who they are and how they came to be that way—a personal and professional biography. As one woman wrote: 'The first place to start should be with myself'. However, as stories of professional practice unfold, a process of recovering oneself by recounting the personal and socio-cultural history behind the stories becomes necessary. The process of reclaiming a personal and professional history involves locating the myths that have shaped our professional life. We may well continue to endorse some of these myths through our practices, even though we pay lip service to rationally constructed theories. Although many myths are identified and rejected, it is apparent that sometimes we replace one myth with another—equally indefensible, except to others who also subscribe to its maintenance. Such distortions and thinking have occurred as nurses react to, rather than reflect upon, the injustices and structured oppression they have experienced from the medical profession. Journal accounts can reveal mythical thinking and provide a place for reflection to proceed.

Journals as revealers of hegemonic practices

Reading practical and theoretical accounts can provide clarification and encouragement to leave the comparative safety of the 'straight and narrow', with its adherence to the 'tried and true', and strike out on a broader, winding path with no immediate end in sight. Courage can be taken from other travellers on the broader, winding path who have written about the experience practically and theoretically. An experienced nurse who interviewed the mother of a patient to find out if the practices on the ward were meeting their demands, wrote in her journal:

> I think the focus on the clinical condition is manifested in the lack of support provided for the parents when they take their kids home. As they are in plaster casts, their clinical condition is stabilised and not a worry, until at least the next visit. What the quality of the experience the parents have at home is not a concern. It is not a concern that someone like Heather stays at home for ten weeks, because she has neither a pram or car seat (which will hold the child in plaster) with which to transport her child anywhere. So she is forced to stay home. Is it any wonder that she is angry. But as this does not have implications for the successful treatment of the clinical condition, to the 'busy' professional it is not a major concern. So Heather is left alone and isolated. On the next visit to outpatients she steps back into the world which is defined by, and has its concern with, the clinical condition. Her experiences, feelings, anger, worries are negated and she's 'kicked out the door'. The situation's constructed to ensure *her* powerlessness and dependency.
>
> Foucault talks about the relationship of knowledge and power. I must read further on this…Another frequent complaint is the absolute inadequacy of information that they are given in hospital. The instrumental reductionist intent, reduces the issue to one of clinical focus…The quality of the experiences of the participants, the mothers and children, comes a poor second best.

As this nurse moves from the descriptive journal account and locates the issue of powerlessness experienced by this mother, she looks to the literature to inform her. She identifies the work of Foucault (1980) on power and knowledge and uses it to view the relationships between participatory power and clinical knowledge. She discovers that the reductionist approach, which narrows the problem to clinical terms, locates power with the professional group, and renders the group who have no knowledge in the clinical area (the parents) powerless. In this way her personal and professional research into her nursing practices through journalling is informed and challenged by her theoretical reading.

Journalling as a collaborative research process

The impetus to keep a journal, when the issues and assumptions which are being revealed challenge cherished, habitual theories and practices, is often the presence of a collaborative relationship. It is not necessary that this person(s) be keeping a journal too, but it is essential that they provide another view of the world in a caring, supportive way. Many nurses, required to journal for their nursing courses, have talked about the support of a partner who is prepared to listen, encourage and challenge taken for granted and distorted views of reality. For others, the comments provided by the course supervisor can provide encouragement, analysis and balance. However, the most appropriate support comes from colleagues who are actively participating in journalling. These relationships can be between people working in very disparate settings but who share a common professional culture. The process of exchanging common themes and issues of concern from their journals enables colleagues to discover the mutuality of their experiences and support each other in developing a collaborative critique of irrational and unjust practices. According to Tracey, a community health nurse:

What an amazing experience reading Joanne's journal. Why so amazing? When I think about it I can see that I expected her concerns to be very different from mine. I probably felt superior to her because I am in community health where we have so much more autonomy and responsibility than someone like her in busy medical ward in that hospital.

What she wrote about—her stories—were very different from mine—they brought back all I want to forget about my hospital nursing days. But when she stood back from them she was working with the same issues as me:

- making sense of the changing nursing role, and
- issues of power and control.

It really is amazing that I thought my issues would be different from hers. It shows me that nurses are still facing the same issues in different ways in different places.

Joanne's journal also reminded me of some of the good things that hospital nurses do. I left because I couldn't stand the problems with the hierarchy. Nurses are always putting each other down, and since I have been working out of the hospital setting I tend to forget the good things that nurses do there—and the good things I did! I am looking forward to talking with Joanne about these things and seeing what sense she made of my journal.

At the time of writing Tracey had just begun a collaborative relationship with Joanne. As the relationship continued it became important as a form of support and encouragement, but it also served to challenge false assumptions about nursing which developed from their personal and situation specific experiences of their own nursing practice. It was apparent in the account when Tracey described the distortion which had developed in her mind in relation to hospital nurses. Although she had rejected the problems of hierarchy in the hospital, she was contributing to the situation by placing community health nurses above hospital nurses. A couple of months later this became apparent to her:

As I look back over what I have written since I started this journal, it has just occurred to me that much of what I write is about problems that other people in the local government hierarchy create for me by their use of power. But now, because of Joanne, I can see that I am playing that game too. I expected that her concerns would be less sophisticated than mine because I saw her, as a hospital nurse, as inferior to the glamour of community health. Then when I realised that she wasn't inferior and she shares my concerns, I decided that she was different to other hospital nurses. I wrote 'Joanne is so different from the usual hospital nurses, she would be good in community health'. How patronising it reads now. I can see that I wanted to hold on to my prejudices about hospital nurses so I made Joanne an exception in my mind. I was playing the hierarchy game which I am always condemning others for!

The collaborative relationship which has developed between these two nurses facilitates the process of personal and professional journalling as research. Continuing collaborative critique enables them to uncover distorted meanings, false assumptions and the gap between rhetoric and reality in their nursing practice.

Posing the problems of practice

As distorted meanings and false assumptions are revealed, the individual's understanding of their reality changes. They begin to see that the questions which they had been busily answering are no longer relevant. As one nurse wrote in her journal:

Tuesday

Now what do I do? This self-rostering has fallen in a big heap. It takes me longer to fix up the messes than it did when I did it myself—and there are still as many complaints. What did I do wrong? The nurses on this ward wanted more autonomy and responsibility. I want to give more to them—self-rostering does this so why isn't it working? I feel that the nurses are not even trying to make it work. Do I give it up altogether?

OK—let's review what I have done. I responded to their dissatisfactions with rostering by deciding to introduce self-rostering. I spent hours of my own time working out the system. I called a staff meeting and explained it all carefully. Everyone was enthusiastic. We started doing it and straight away things went wrong...

Thursday

I wrote it all out and then had to leave it. Now when I re-read what I wrote I can suddenly see 'I', 'I', 'I' everywhere! I wasn't handing over power and responsibility. I was just changing the rules that they had to follow. Now where does that get me? I must admit I don't really know what the nurses want in the way of rostering. I never really asked them except in a general way. We all presumed that self-rostering was a good thing and we all assumed that I had the power to design and enforce it. I thought the answer to the question 'how do I transfer some power and responsibility to the staff' was to introduce self-rostering. I thought I had the answer but now I am not even sure that I understand the question. So what do I do now—well perhaps I should rephrase it to what shall *we* do? Yes that's it! I will start by talking about autonomy and responsibility and perhaps *we* can come up with the right answers.

Through journalling this nurse has been confronted with the implications of her controlling actions and has come to recognise that she can't force autonomy and responsibility onto others. Her journal reveals the manner in which her language reflects her unacknowledged practices. She decides that she has assumed the question to be answered. As this question has remained implicit, she finds that she is no longer sure that she is asking the right question. However at this stage she still wants to move from an issue of autonomy and responsibility through an implicit question to the 'right answers'. However, as her journal demonstrates a week later, this understanding is challenged through her reflection on the meeting.

Well that meeting was really illuminating. I wrote last week that perhaps WE can come up with the right answers. It seems that the most important issue is hierarchical control—and I have been busily maintaining that—but it is evident from today's meeting that we needn't bother about the answers as we haven't even begun to ask the right questions—at least not any that can be answered. It is exciting—but scary too. Sympathised with Jean when she said, 'Wasn't it easier when we all followed orders and knew exactly what to do?' Well I have opened up the can of worms now so I will have to work with the others to work out what to do next. I must admit I liked the feeling that we were in this together and it wasn't me against them as I have often felt before.

Through the collaborative interaction with her colleagues and through her journal reflection, this nurse has moved from a position of working with assumed questions and predictable answers, to a position where even the questions are acknowledged as unknown. In the process this nurse is moving between the realities and constraints of the actual situation to the freedom of the possible. She is beginning to open up the issue so that new and appropriate questions can be posed—questions which are explicit and grounded in her newly espoused theory that nurses need to work together to develop strategies that change the rules of the power game.

Making new perspectives

The process of journalling is a process of change. As descriptive accounts are collected and analysed the values, theories, attitudes and assumptions in use in professional practice are exposed. The exposure leads to reflection on the person as a professional and on the socio-cultural situation. Over time a narrative account emerges which transcends the 'now' of the present and reaches into the 'then' of the past to inform and interpret personal and professional development. These forays into the past illuminate the present and provide challenges to future action. Change is inevitable. Change in understanding leads to changes in action. The journal provides a record of these changes, which challenge and encourage, however it is not always a comfortable process. As one nurse wrote:

I am fed up with everything—particularly with keeping this journal. Do I do it to have a record of my failures? If I hadn't started writing then I wouldn't have been aware of all these things I want to change. What was I thinking of when I started writing six months ago?

How incredible! I have just re-read all my journal. Was that really me? I thought I had done nothing much in that time but now I am amazed at what I've done. Some of those things I wrote at the beginning, I cringe at now—but I must admit there were some important things written there too. I liked what I wrote about the need to change. It was good—I can hardly believe that I wrote it. And the success of introducing those changes to hand over procedures. That was a good change—it has really worked—even if it took me a few tries to get it right. I have marked those pages so that I can find them easily. I need to revisit them and remind myself of what we have achieved since we began this journey together—my journal and I. Now where do we go from here, journal? Perhaps if I start by writing down the things that are really bugging me at the moment I may be able to get them into some sort of perspective.

The documentation of changed understandings, the recording of action and its consequences, and the reflections upon these, are elements which enable the writer to move beyond the subjective feelings of the moment. The feeling self is transformed into a spectator and analyst of his or her own personal professional drama. Journals supply the raw data for this kind of examination and the process by which it can occur. As journal keepers change their practices to reflect more accurately the personal and professional philosophies which they espouse, their journals provide them with the opportunity to reflect systematically upon these changes, and their consequences, for the individual and the situation; and to examine the resulting changes in their understanding. The systematic recording enables the changes to be analysed in accordance with those issues which the changes were designed to address.

Embodiment as a limit to change

The concept of embodiment and the effects of our learnt body patterns upon our capacity to change, and facilitate change, is an area which becomes apparent upon reading journal narratives. However the very taken for grantedness of our embodiment as persons and workers means that the area is often neglected by journal keepers. It is a concept which I only became fully aware of in my own journal after keeping it for a number of years. During a research project when I was required to follow and document the work of busy clinical nurses, I soon discovered the difference in the disciplines which had been imposed upon my body from theirs. I wrote:

Oh my aching legs!! My body has forgotten what it is like to be on my feet all day. These nurses are so used to it, they assume that I am fine following them everywhere, being jammed into corners or left to stand for long periods of time. My work role has involved a lot more time sitting—in meetings, at my desk, at my computer, with staff and clients. Most lectures I give at least provide me with a lectern to lean on and only take an hour or so. Others are conducted around tables so it is a case of sitting down again. So I find it hard to continue concentrating on data collection when I am dying to sit down and have a cup of coffee. And speaking of food and drink I am used to eating much less and drinking more during my working day. These women fuel their work activities with dim sims and enormous coffee scrolls at 9.45 in the morning! Even after a small breakfast at 6.15 a.m. there is no way I can face that kind of food three hours later. But I do miss the mugs of coffee—with staff, clients, during meetings and especially when I am writing. My eating habits have been fine for my sedentary role but they are not working very well for me now in this context. I am an embodied being whose patterns no longer fit my current work patterns. Yet, as this is only a temporary situation, I don't really want to change—modify a bit but not change—or I will end up the size of an elephant.

I can see now how embodiment is really a limit to change. I must read about this more—retrospectively in my journals—and in the literature on embodiment and rational change.

Pursuing this concept of embodiment through my own journal, and with nurses through their journals, enabled me to recognise the place of embodiment in the process of journal keeping. As a result of my journal account of embodiment I was able to research both my own practices and those of other journal keepers in relation to this issue. I already had plenty of raw data for analysis in my collection of journal accounts. I found that some nurses, who have been trained to stand and to focus on oral communication, can find writer's blocks when required to sit down and write about their activities. The insight was particularly helpful for some nurses who, in a discussion session, explained that they had felt guilty because they found it difficult to sit and write. Upon analysing their work days, we discovered that most of their brief writing tasks were done quickly on their feet. This understanding led some nurses to decide to begin writing while they were doing other habitual mechanical tasks at home, as that often started the recall and thinking process flowing. Later they would relax and sit down to work further with their journals since it coincided with their normal routine of sitting down after the evening meal. This recognition of the role embodiment plays in their professional practices enabled these nurses to develop journalling practices which were in accordance with their habitual patterns of physical work and leisure.

It is apparent that the journal provides an ongoing data base—a rich resource which can be revisited and analysed in new ways as new insights and knowledge develop. When new questions are posed, the same accounts can be revisited and provide different knowledge depending on the focus of the question.

Journalling as a reflective process

The ongoing data base provided by a personal and professional journal provides not only information on the content of professional practice, but on the process of reflection itself. In this way the journal provides a process for meta-theorising—thinking about the processes of thinking. This is evident when individuals revisit their experiences and examine the ways in which they constructed their thinking at the time of the account. A nurse who had kept a journal of her nursing actions over twelve months concluded:

As I read over my journal for the year I noticed three main things—

1. My assumptions, attitudes and actions have changed. Well that's not too surprising. When I finally had the courage to begin to journal I already knew that it had this 'change' effect from what had happened to a couple of other nurses I know.
2. My knowledge and understanding has changed—another ho-hum. Well of course it would wouldn't it?
3. My understanding of how I 'know' things and how I learn things has changed. This is harder to explain but I can see how my limited view of knowledge came from my nursing *training*—it certainly wasn't education! When I look through the journal at the way I wrote things at the beginning and the way I write now—it isn't just that I know more but that I 'know' differently. I have moved beyond an automatic, cause and effect way of thinking into a way of understanding that—well I don't really know how to describe it properly yet but I know it is different. I think more about issues and analyse things for myself rather than leaving that to other people. Even trying to write about this shows that I have moved miles from the beginning when I wrote things like:
'Looked after Mr. T. Nice man. Told me about his daughter when I did his obs—she is a travel agent—always on the move—sounds like a good job! Makes me wonder why I am stuck here wiping old men's bums!'

I feel much better about myself—deeper somehow—and I can see that there is a change in the way I nurse—I am more creative and responsive, more responsible too.

This journal entry demonstrates the progression made from simple to complex forms of self-reflection. They not only represent processes of knowing but include reflection on the processes of changing action. As one nurse wrote:

> As I reflect on where I have come this year with my journal I can see…in recent times my outlook has changed and I therefore feel that I can state that I *am* able to change. I would like to start taking control of my professional nursing life by:
>
> - standing by my convictions
> - being prepared to state an opinion even though it may conflict with that of my superiors/common group. This means being sure in my own mind just what my opinions/philosophies are, because I am sure that they need an overhaul given the fact that they have not received correct use for a long time—if ever.
>
> But if I can manage to do these things I think the benefits will be many, not the least being the personal value of an increase (and a much needed one) in self-esteem.

This nurse recognises that her former ways of thinking and acting were no longer appropriate—and that they had never been very helpful to her as demonstrated by her lack of self-esteem. She is prepared to examine her opinions and philosophies and then to own them in discussions with others. She sees the reflective process of journalling as a means of developing her input into debates with others, an area she neglected.

Journalling as a political act

A word of warning—journalling is never a neutral process. Journalling is a political process. Through reflection the power of the individual to engage in individual and collaborative actions with political intent is revealed (Kemmis 1985). These actions occur within a sociocultural framework of meaning which both constructs and defines them. Therefore it is never an apolitical process as some people would like to claim. According to one nurse:

> I'm a little hesitant about delving deeply. Surely there is a lot to be said about ignorance being bliss. Maintaining the status quo and not rocking the boat is worth considering. I'm an apolitical kind of nurse. I just go along and do my job.

The daily rituals we engage in to maintain the prevailing structures of our day to day lives are political acts. An 'apolitical kind of nurse' acts politically by engaging in deliberate inaction that maintains the status quo. However inaction is not always this passive accommodation to the dominant cultural practices. Keeping a journal may disclose the power of transformative inaction— another kind of inaction which challenges controlling practices. Such deliberate inaction facilitates power sharing, enabling others to participate in the issues and decisions which affect their daily lives. One nurse writes:

I am just beginning to let go and let the patients make more choices in their own time and in their own way. It has been hard. I had to learn *not* to do things for them that they could do for themselves. This holding back is becoming a constant theme in my journal.

Journalling is a reflective process which enables the development of a personal and professional identity with the capacity to deconstruct the relationships between thought and action, knowledge and practice, values and assumptions, and the individual and society.

A final warning—keeping a journal can become addictive.

9. Living the research experience

Nursing literature is replete with pleas for the development of clinical nursing research. Many people speak about it, teach about it, write about it and encourage others to do it. Few people do clinical nursing research and fewer engage in praxis processes. This chapter is dedicated to people who, like me, have embarked upon the risky business of actually engaging in reflective praxis and feminist processes in the context of nursing practice. I have tried to put forward the voices of participatory nurse researchers speaking about their own experiences.

The role of the participatory researcher is often fraught with anxiety as reflection discloses the competing positions of oneself as researcher—one minute accountable to ethics committees and the funding agency, the next minute a participant in the problem formulation or data collection, the next the organiser of functional supports such as meeting times, spaces, storage, and equipment maintenance, and the next the person reflecting on the power relations inherent in all these activities and how the opportunities to exercise power affect the direction of the research. Discussion on the role of the researcher among the action research community ranges from structuring the role as facilitator to full participant. Nurse action researchers have discussed this in terms of the role of facilitator, and focused on what East and Robinson (1994) describe as management of change. Other nurses have worked together in the action research process with access to a researcher as a guide and critical friend (Goulding 1993, Kennedy 1993, McEwan 1993). Some action research groups have a researcher as a full participating member (Robinson et al 1993, McClelland et al 1993). I seem to have taken on at times all these roles and have found that I constantly needed to negotiate reflexively with the participants and continually reflect on my own exercise of power.

I would like to explore briefly some of the tensions and dilemmas which arise for nurses as researchers of their own practise and for participatory researchers working with them.

The value of participatory research for nurses

When a varied group of nurses were asked the question, 'What is nursing research?' there were varied responses which included:

Nurses doing research about their own practice. Has to be done by nurses and needs to have an action component that can be implemented.

Nursing research is effecting change on practice and beneficial to practice, but it may not always be related specifically to the patients.

More nursing related as opposed to anatomical and physical sort of research.

Nursing research...well one thing, [is that] nurses are doing it. Research is not necessarily finding out the answers but finding out possibilities. Understanding the area you're researching better, and that understanding allows you to make more informed decisions. It allows you to be more creative and more lateral in your thinking. You're able to implement new ideas that you come up with. And then, probably an evaluation.

These answers show that many nurses believe increased understanding and changed practice is a desirable outcome of research activities. PAR is a valuable method for nurses interested in examining the areas of concern to them in their day to day lives and then acting to modify or change those areas. It provides a framework by which individuals can join with their friends or colleagues to improve the situation for themselves and on behalf of others. One nurse explained her position:

I get very disheartened, we do a lot of work to change things, and then look to see that nothing becomes of it. I think that with action research we can have a change for the better, or even make people more aware of the situation. For example, I did a discharge survey on the unit. [It was] very small, [I did it because] the staff kept saying to me, 'We're always the last one to know when the patient's to go home. The doctor always tells us last.' So for two or three months I surveyed every patient that went home. And the results were that 70% of staff were the first people to be told. So, it showed me that what they were telling me was wrong.

This nurse was able to confirm that what was being constantly reported to her was exaggerated. However as she conducted the survey she uncovered the reasons staff were feeling they were uninformed. She concluded that her research:

also highlighted what some of the problems were. So I can't bear to see information being done and gathered and just sitting there in dust. It has to be brought back out for people to see, even if it's just information, and knowledge.

Commitment to research

Although the motivation to engage in research is for some nurses allied with further development of their professional practice, for others it becomes necessary as a form of accountability in the climate created by tight budgets. When the motivation comes from external pressures and not interest and a desire to learn and grow professionally, the commitment is often minimal. One nurse reported:

We saw that on our own ward, the people who participated in the research, learnt and grew [whereas] the people that didn't—well, they didn't! They didn't learn and they didn't grow personally or professionally probably, as much as what we did.

Another nurse explained how the confidence in her professional growth through the research process enabled her to deal with a challenging situation:

It was quite interesting. The ward was going to close down to amalgamate, and it was then [I heard] that people's names were going to be drawn out of a hat [to see] who stays on the ward...And I said, 'Forget it, this is my career. I'm not having my name drawn out of a hat. We go for an interview for a position, like you normally would.' I said, 'I don't have a problem with that, I believe I have something to offer this ward', and my colleagues said, 'Oh...' And I said, 'Well what can you offer?' and they answered 'Well, I don't know'. And I said, 'Well, you should be thinking about what you're giving to this ward. It's OK, you just do the normal nursing task, but you need to be learning and growing and stuff.'

This nurse's challenge to some of her colleagues had an effect. She and others in her research group had been trying to get staff to document their experiences at managing a specific condition. When the staff understood that they may be expected to demonstrate their knowledge and commitment in an interview, their research productivity increased. She continued:

It was amazing, by the end of that week, when we thought we were going to have interview—we never did—I had about ten [research] accounts being written, because people decided, 'Well, this looks good', and, 'This is going to help me', and all that. So people don't always do things for the right reasons.

This nurse's insight about many people doing the right thing for the wrong reason helped her to think over what it takes to change people's attitudes:

But it wasn't a real change in attitude. I would have hoped it was. I mean there's nothing wrong [with what they did]. They've got to save their job. But, I mean, changing peoples attitudes, you need to go through this long slow process.

There are many reasons good nurses do not become involved in research. Nurses who are involved in further studies or work part time with other responsibilities at home may provide excellent care during their time on the ward but not want to participate in something which requires attention after hours. One nurse said:

There are also the nurses that come to work, do their work, and go home. You've got to accept that. And while they're here for their seven and a half hours, eight hours, they're actually at work, they give 100% in their clinical care of the kids, but they don't do any more than that. And there are still some nurses out there that do not get heavily involved in anything no matter what.

When nurses are enthusiastic about research they can find it difficult to accept that some of their peers will always be un-interested. Sometimes this apathy relates to an attitude about nursing as, 'The work that pays the school fees, that's all I do it for'. On the other hand for some of these nurses the time is not right to take on the extra commitment. As one nurse explained:

I only work part-time and come home to three small children, one starting school, one starting kinder and the other one in playgroup, and they are good kids but they run me ragged, and...They have health problems so we have specialist's appointments and [I find it hard] just trying to do everything. I really like these old people. I enjoy 'me work'. I can focus on the needs of my patients, but after work well I go back to it all. That's all I can manage right now.

Another nurse who had been a very valuable member of an action research project during one year recognised that her priorities were different the following year:

I am doing my honors and I wanted to get involved in the research like I was last year. But then I had to do a research project for my honors and it was all too much.

Participatory research is demanding and requires commitment. It means that staff need to set different priorities and be prepared to work on the research in their own time. However most staff find that their research activities are rewarding and beneficial both personally and professionally.

The benefits of research

Many nurses think about their research experience and see it as valuable for their own knowledge and practice and for the unit where they work:

The more research that goes on in a ward, the more conducive the environment is to research, and the more people are willing to take it on and are actually interested in trying to improve their clinical practice and issues that are outstanding, that are a problem or an interest to them.

Another nurse noticed that there were changes in practice which the group attributed to their study:

Because we were doing the research over such a long period of time, we did notice changes on the ward, and we feel it was a result of our study. People became quite interested in what we were doing, and the issues that we were raising as the study went on. Basically the research came up with all these really good ways and strategies to overcome some of the procedures that we were doing, like changing procedures. And it also changed some of the people in the group's attitudes about the issue and how we were dealing with it.

Another benefit which was often mentioned by nurses who had participated in clinical research was their increased participation in education programs. For example:

I know there's a lot of interest in our ward. We've got about 20 to 25 staff and everybody's very, very involved in something, a degree, or if not study outside [the hospital] then the paediatric course or diabetic education, things like that.

I have found that there is a very high proportion of nurses who have been involved in participatory research who go on to do specialist and graduate courses. Many nurses attribute a growth in the self-esteem and confidence to attempt further education to the knowledge and skills that they gained in research.

Nurses were also able to identify other own professional gains from engaging in research. One clinical nurse was able to get a research assistant job because of her work on the unit's project. She described the experience as:

Honestly, I wouldn't feel...like I said before, I'm on this really steep learning curve. But I wouldn't feel...as in tune, if you like, if I hadn't done that research. And that's not from a professional point of view, like from getting a job, but from a personal point of view. It's a real growth time for me.

She was able to remark about the personal cost that she carried at the time:

It was hard, and mostly your own time, and I wouldn't (have) given it up for anything, 'cause I really, really learnt about what I was doing and stuff, and it gave me...it gives me now, much more confidence, if I see something wrong, to go in and say, 'Hey, I mightn't know the answer, but that's not right what you're doing, and we really need to look at this'.

Other nurses recognised the value of the research relationships which develop in participatory research projects:

So...yeah it was great. And I...yeah, the people that were in the group, you sort of really bond with them...I mean I haven't seen...J for ages, you know, but...there's just this feeling that you went through all this together.

Changing nursing culture through research

Looking beyond individual gains permitted some nurses to see how the culture in the ward changed with nurses being involved in the research process. One reported:

I actually think that the research that we did before this project was more difficult. Well within our ward anyway, research, sort or started about three years ago, and I think when it first started, people were quite anxious about it, and there was a lot of animosity towards people who were involved in research by the other people, because they saw the research as not being important. They saw it, as...a waste of time, and they saw it really as something that wasn't productive or useful. But as the research has sort of taken over...they've noticed changes within a ward environment, Then I have heard some of these people saying that it can be quite a useful tool for exploring issues, and then coming up, sometimes, with better solutions.

Single projects can occur without having much effect on the culture of the ward. However, when a number of small groups can function, the unit staff begin to see changes and participation rates improve dramatically. Participatory projects are very useful in this way because they are localised and relevant and have feedback loops which enable pragmatic nurses to see the effects of the research activity.

But I think within our ward, because we've been exposed to so much research over the years, I think the environment's certainly changed, and people are certainly more receptive to what goes on, and to joining in, and to being interested in it. Originally people were very skeptical, and they'd question you in a very negative way. Now, they're really interested in what you're doing.

This situation is also true in academic settings. It is very difficult to develop a research culture in a university nursing school when the emphasis is on teaching and administration. There needs to be a critical mass of staff engaging in research before the priorities, attitudes and work practices change to support research as an everyday activity for academic nurses.

Another nurse spoke of the cultural change in her ward as a result of the work by the clinical researcher and the staff. She saw the clinical researcher as a key resource person for the group:

I think the main issue about how research has been useful, is of cultural change... for nurses themselves, and I think that we had a lot of problems initially with action research because the people that were doing [it] didn't really understand the process. You know, we'd have J [the researcher] there chatting, and J was enthusiastic about it all, and she was learning a lot about it, too, and I mean, nurses are great. We're in among it.

However the clinical or teaching demands experienced by nurse researchers mean that a research culture is still an adjunct to other activities rather than being a central activity. A researcher noted:

Our whole culture is, it still is, that we're there, not for research. We're there to look after the patients, and time and time again we would miss research meetings saying, 'I can't go, I've got to do this for my patient...We don't have any time to leave the ward.' And it's...various wards have this attitude. It's part of the culture.

Nurses may find that the adage 'for the good of the patient' is also a good excuse not to engage in other activities such as research because the patient's best interests are always assumed to be related to ceaseless activity rather than to other professional activities of research and reading. The culture of busyness means that nurses may feel guilty if they are not doing things for the patient and yet many of the activities are administrative. In this culture nurses may provide expert care for their patients but not for themselves, or for their colleagues, as is evident in the following account of the change in attitude of one nurse who has been involved in research:

It's not only just the nursing culture. Various wards have different cultures, I mean, my partner works on another ward, and they have this total commitment to care in which...well, we on our ward do too, but it, it really shines out to me on their ward—'For the Patient'—so much so, that I don't think they care for each other. So when it comes to the end of the day at three, or three thirty, on our ward, I think we do care for each other. We say 'Oh, go, come on, you've done your bit today, get off the ward, go home. Cause it's a high stress area, and you need to relax.' and I go off to pick up my partner, and it'll be 4 o'clock and she's still answering phones. And I just put my hand on the phone and say, 'Look, you know...', and it's [she slaps me]. What I'm trying to say is, I mean, the cultures are all so inbuilt on each ward, depending on who the management head is. But I think the over all culture is that we can't leave our patients or the phones. So therefore, if you can somehow, and I don't know...the answer. We've been struggling for years. I think it is a bit better. I think we do...um...make time now for research, we see the value of it for the care of everyone. But...the only reason...it's a pretty harsh comment...I really believe the only reason that it happens on our ward is because we've got a unit manager that says, 'Right, you're doing research today'. If it was left up to the people themselves, they wouldn't have gone, they wouldn't you know. I mean, if it wasn't for her we probably wouldn't do any. I mean, she's given us these days to go off and do it. And I think the majority of industries and professions out there do support research like that. But I don't think there's many unit managers in the hospital like ours, that actually support research as much.

So a cultural change is necessary if a group of people are going to change their habitual practices and to value participatory research activities. This cultural change can be very challenging for staff from other places where research is not given the same priority and they may react defensively by attacking the value of research for clinicians. Nurse who participate in praxis research may have to defend their involvement to their peers who often want to have instant results demonstrated to them.

So, I mean, that's...there if I was to, sort of push for a change in culture, then the unit managers are the people that I would be directing the main push to, and not just on one ward. I went to a unit manager's meeting, oh, it must have been...almost a year and a half ago, and they were all talking about this action research, and said to me, 'Oh, it seems ridiculous', and they were really getting stuck into [criticising] it, and I said, 'Ah, what do you actually know about it?' 'Oh, well, you know, it's a waste of time, and blah blah blah blah', and they really went to town, and I said, 'Well, you know, we do it on our ward and I think it's pretty good, actually'. And they said, 'Well, what do you know about it?' And I said, 'Well, I still don't know the full thing'. And so I just get a little bit amazed that people start slagging off at something they don't actually know anything about. It's not threatening or anything like that. I said, 'It's done some good things on the ward, changed our practice a little bit'. 'Oh, but you know, it takes so long, and you don't get any results'. And I said, 'Well, I would argue that we do get results. We function better as a ward because of...a lot of the action research. We've changed things we've been trying to change for years, as opposed to someone coming in and saying, "You've got to do this now"'. This way you do it yourselves by just going through a cycle, 'Oh well, we're going to do this now', and get on with it.

For units where the culture includes nursing research as part of professional activity the enthusiasm and interest is often high and the contributions of all staff are valued. One enthusiastic nurse commented:

I find that nurses at the bedside make great contributions to research, and like, their knowledge and that sort of thing would be really valuable to try and tap into. I sort of feel that there's a lot of untapped people just working at the beds that would be fantastic just to involve in research more. So although you would never expect to incorporate everyone into it, but...just to give everyone the opportunity if they want to...

This nurse generates a very positive attitude about research activities and the potential contributions of her peers. When nurses generate enthusiasm about research like this they can facilitate the involvement of others. Another enthusiastic nurse commented:

Nursing research is something that is just beginning really. Like it's been going on for a while, but it's really getting to a point now where it's really making a difference. It's really good. And I think the more nurses that work with research, the more research comes out of the ward, the more willing they are to participate in it when they see that all can contribute [to something] really, beneficial But it is quite exciting to go to do something and then see a change or become more enlightened as a result of it. And once people have gone down that path and seen that, I think they're all keen to do it again. 'Cause did you note that T wanted to do another research project? And then other people get interested, and think, 'Oh, that sounds really good', so then they join in as well. And certainly you recruit more people as you go along. It's great. Just generating all that interest.

Nurses who have participated in participatory forms of research argue that research should not be an elitist activity reserved for a few privileged nurses, but that the opportunities should be presented to all nurses. One said:

I think it should be an opportunity for everybody...it should be something that's open to all nurses within a clinical session. 'Cause I feel some nurses are probably more interested in research than others, I sort of think that we should be developing research from the bottom up. I mean, we all need to...to learn. I think it's the only way we're going to change nursing, and to examine our own practice and examine where we're coming from, and I think that has to come from, from all levels. I think, if you just made...if you just take it to the nurse managers and educators, it sort of gives it that...not elitist type thing, but it sort of...I mean it just should be made available at all levels. Though I certainly think that people up the ladder should be taking it on as well, but I think it should be within a ward level, open to the...to the registered clinical nurses as well.

There is a need to for nurses to conduct research into the structure of the clinical nursing role in order to better understand and articulate what it is that they do. One nurse talked about this issue as he experienced it:

I've done a tertiary degree in business, and in one of the human resource management classes, we had to outline what we did in our day, and break it up into various things. And I broke my day as an associate charge nurse down with about 80% of my time spent in communicating to staff members and patients families. And they just say, 'That can't be true', because the course was done with other people who didn't really know a lot about nursing. And they said, 'How can you spend 80% of your day…' and they picked me out and said 'Break down your day', and, 'What you?' And went through it all, and this guy said, 'Well, you obviously have a fairly good idea of what you do during your day', and I said, 'Well, that's just it, I don't think the majority of nurses do'. I said, 'I can tell you all those things', and I said, 'But my day's like everyone else's'. He said, 'How can you spend 80% of your day talking?' and I said, 'It's not just talking, it's listening, and communicating and making people feel comfortable'. We don't tend to value that, and I don't think it gets valued a lot by a lot of other people either. If we don't understand what we do we can't see how to incorporate research into it.

The challenges for the career nursing researcher

Although engaging in research brings its own special pressures and challenges for nurses who are employed in a clinical, educational or administrative role, there are a different but equally demanding set of issues for career researchers who use praxis processes with nurses.

Dealing in uncertainties

Embarking upon these types of research processes indicates that we have reached a crisis of confidence in the prevailing order with its separation of the researcher from the researched. The pursuit of participatory processes is a risky business because the researcher is in a vulnerable position. No longer can the researcher hide his or her own subjectivity behind an objective facade of research procedures built up by categorising people as sample populations—statistics—which have to be investigated in ways that are reliable and replicate the procedures used to investigate natural phenomena. The participatory researcher has to negotiate the research to take account of the power relationships and hierarchies that can be constructed within the research process. The researcher has to be able to meet the challenge of activities which value reciprocity and collaboration and collegiality and changing subject positions. Participatory researchers engage in a process which is always open to contestation. It is a process in which the participatory researcher is unable to control the research activities, the research meanings or the outcomes because these things are all shared and negotiated with the research participants.

As researchers we are often naive and over enthusiastic. We generally engage in research because we want answers to questions that concern or interest us. If we reject more orthodox research methods for the challenges of participatory research, we do so because we have a commitment to maintaining particular research values. But we may want our research to do too much. We engage in a diligent search for certainties in the same way as more orthodox researchers search for facts. We find ourselves faced with multiple theoretical and methodological positions which require us to pose new questions and search for new answers. We find difficult problems with no obvious answers or with many alternative answers. We find we need to keep justifying our methods in the light of our research values and their rhetoric. And if we are honestly engaging in critical reflection on our praxis processes, we find ourselves with doubts, dilemmas and sometimes despair over our role as researcher.

Doubts arise when we begin to understand the limits of our theoretical and methodological bases. When this happens we can begin to doubt ourselves as researchers. We have invested so much in a new way of thinking and acting, that we don't want to doubt theory and methodology. It is easier to lose confidence and accept that there is something wrong with us when our research demonstrates the limitations of our theory, or our understandings of our theory. When this happens, it usually means that, although we name ourselves 'critical' or 'feminist' or 'praxis-oriented' or 'post structuralist', we are acting as if theory and practice are totally separate, and as if right theory can be applied as right practice. We need to acknowledge the cyclic or spiral nature of praxis research with its ongoing interplay between understanding, reflection and action. This means that if something doesn't work as we expected, the reflective process allows us to analyse the changed situation and the new meanings which we create out of this process. The theory of participatory research also charges us with the task of reflecting on the way we exercise power as researchers in the process, and the effect of this activity on the situation and our own understandings. That thinking then informs our changed actions. This is the PAR rhetoric. However, as Carson (1990) and his colleagues discovered, the rhetoric of critically reflective action research suggests that it is possible to scrutinise objectively the subjective interpretations of the participants to reach a critical understanding through transformative action. The difficulties they encountered in making this a reality sent them back to their interpretive position, and they argue for a 'hermeneutics of practice' (Carson 1990:173).

However those of us who are influenced by post structuralist or post modern thinking are 'suspicious' of both a hermeneutics of practice and critical reflection (Ellsworth 1989) as being limited by the discourses in which they were formed—a process described as 'troubling' by Patti Lather (1993). She argues that as feminist and critical methods of research 'trouble' the explanations based on understanding, so post modern deconstruction 'troubles' the answers provided by critical and some feminist reflective processes and is troubled in return by them.

When we work in this way we may still find that the process leads to self-doubt. It is important to realise that self-doubt is frequent for the researcher who is forging new paths. Accountability as a researcher not only rests on the product produced, that is the research, but also on the processes, and the effects on others and on the situation. When the focus dwells on the self the researcher is not using his or her social imagination but is locked into an individualistic form of psychotherapy. This difference is crucial. Through our social imagination we identify and acknowledge the particular circumstances, structures and understandings which contribute to what is perceived as problematic. We begin by blending individual stories and visions into collaborative ones.

Conundrums arise as we struggle to find words reflect our changing understandings and agendas. Deconstructing and changing our language, however, does not resolve the original dilemmas of engaging in the research processes. New language does, however, enable us to think about our actions in new ways, which in turn enable us to uncover the unacknowledged, taken for granted assumptions which inform our socio-cultural views.

The process of questioning our language confronts the symbols and images which are expressed in the habitual language we use. The attainment of new language removes issues from the domain of their dominant discourse and locates them in an alternative discourse which is not legitimated by institutional nursing structures. The construction of an alternate discourse of nursing is a lonely position for a nurse by definition. As we struggle to identify and change the symbols and images which constitute the dominant discourse we discover that our understanding, and the understandings of our colleagues, are being challenged.

Confronting ourselves as researchers

Looking honestly at themselves is never a comfortable process for individuals or groups. If we engage in this kind of confrontation of ourselves, our myths and our practices, we generally have a crisis of confidence. Although it almost seems inevitable, it is encouraging to know that the crisis is part of the pain of genuine development. It is also encouraging to make that journey with others—preferably others who have also experienced and survived the pain in some small way. It is the nature of critical reflection to undo the defensive beliefs that are socially constructed and endorsed, freeing us to search for alternative ways of thinking and imaging the world through language.

However at this point it is important to remind ourselves that we are not ethereal sources of discourse capable of transcending our bodies and their somatic history. Fay (1987:146) obliges us to recognise that 'oppression leaves its traces not just in people's minds, but in their muscles and skeletons as well'.

The understanding of the interrelationship between our will, our desires, our experience and our bodies is essential in engaging in critical reflection. Despair arises when we find that our quest to understand and improve practice is limited by our embodiment and those things that it is not possible for us to think because of the discourses we inhabit. We discover that we are not capable of being fully rational and disinterested in a collaborative search for absolute and universalised, fundamental, moral and political principles. The values which we hold, both consciously and unconsciously, and the ways in which we have thought and acted previously and elsewhere are inscribed upon our bodies. We reap a harvest from the Platonic mind and body split, which our society has been constructed around. We have learnt to see our bodies only as biological cages which hold our inner thinking selves. This is difficult to unlearn. We live our own individual and combined histories. Research provides constant challenges to unpick the experiences.

Like many worthwhile things, establishing research in a clinical nursing context is demanding. After the honeymoon when everyone is keen and things move swiftly, the career researcher needs to deal with the relationship with staff. Their interest is waning because research is time consuming and doesn't give the instant solutions people are looking for.

Different positions in the hierarchy bring different challenges for the career researcher. Some with senior positions find that their role becomes administrative and political—dealing with structures and policies more than people and research data. Other career researchers do not have enough institutional power and can find themselves rapidly absorbed into other related roles such as quality assurance project officers.

Despite all these dilemmas and contradictions participatory research is worth doing. It enables researchers to share in the lives and experiences of others. It creates opportunities for researchers to meet nurses and replay the dramas of nursing practice, working together to solve problems that make a difference. This is a privilege and it is fun.

References

Allen D, Benner P et al 1986 Three paradigms for nursing research: methodological implications. In: Chinn P L (ed) Nursing research methodology: issues and implementation. Aspen, Rockville, Maryland

Allen D G 1985 Nursing research and social control: alternative models of science that emphasize understanding and emancipation. Image: Journal of Nursing Scholarship Spring, 23(2):58-64

Benner P 1984 From novice to expert: excellence and power in clinical nursing practice. Addison-Wesley, California

Benner P, Wrubel J 1989 The primacy of caring. Addison-Wesley, Sydney

Blackford J 1993 Moving towards empowerment. Royal Children's Hospital, Melbourne

Carr W 1989 Action research: ten years on. Journal of Curriculum Studies 21(1):85-90

Carr W, Kemmis S 1986 Becoming critical: knowing through action research. Deakin University Press, Geelong

Carson T 1990 What kind of knowing is critical action research? Theory Into Practice 29(3):167-173

Chaska N 1978 The nursing profession: views through the mist. McGraw-Hill, New York

Chaska N 1983 The nursing profession: a time to speak. McGraw-Hill, New York

Chinn P L 1985 Debunking myths in nursing theory and research. Image: Journal of Nursing Scholarship 23(2):45-49

Chinn P L (ed) 1986 Nursing research methodology: issues and implementation. Aspen, Rockville

Christ C P, Plaskow J 1979 Womanspirit rising. Harper & Row, San Francisco

Chuaprapaisilip A 1990 Improving learning from experience: action research in nursing education in Thailand. First World Congress on Action Research and Process Management. Griffith University, Brisbane

Clarke M 1976 Action and reflection: practice and theory in nursing. Journal of Advanced Nursing 11:3-11

Colomina B (ed) 1992 Sexuality and space. Princeton Architectural Press, New Jersey

Connors D D 1988 A continuum of researcher-participant relationships: an analysis and critique. Journal of Advanced Nursing Science 10(4):32-42

Daly M 1978 Gyn/ecology: the metaethics of radical feminism. Beacon Press, Boston

de Beauvoir S 1961 The second sex (1949). Bantam, New York

de Lauretis T (ed) 1988 Feminist studies/critical studies. Macmillan, Houndsmills

Dunlop M J 1986 Is a science of caring possible? Journal of Advanced Nursing 11:661-670

East L, Robinson J 1994 Change in process: bringing about change in health care through action research. Journal of Clinical Nursing 3:57-61

Ellsworth E 1989 Why doesn't this feel empowering? Working through the repressive myths of critical pedagogy. Harvard Educational Review 59(3):297-324

Fawcett J 1984 Hallmarks of success in nursing research. Advances in Nursing Science 7(1):1-11

Fay B 1977 How people change themselves: the relationship between critical theory and its audience. In: Bull T (ed) Political theory and praxis: new perspectives. University of Minnesota Press, Minnesota

Fay B 1987 Critical social science. Cornell University Press, Ithaca

Fine M 1992 Disruptive voices: the possibilities of feminist research. University of Michigan Press, Ann Arbor

Foster J 1993 Take me to Paris Johnny. Minerva, Port Melbourne

Foucault M 1972 The archeology of knowledge. Tavistock, London

Foucault M 1977 Discipline and punish: the birth of the prison. Pantheon, New York

Foucault M 1977 What is an author? In: Bouchard D F (ed) Language, counter-memory, practice. Cornell University Press, Ithaca, New York

Foucault M 1980 Power and knowledge. In: Gordon G (ed) Selected interviews and other writings. Pantheon, New York

Foucault M 1982 The subject and power. In: Dreyfus H, Rabinow P (eds) Michel Foucault: beyond structuralism and hermeneutics. Harvester Press, Brighton

Fraser N, Nicholson L 1988 Social criticism without philosophy: an encounter between feminism and postmodernism. In: Ross A (ed) Universal abandon: the politics of postmodernism. University of Minnesota Press, Minneapolis 83-104

Freire P 1972 Pedagogy of the oppressed. Penguin, Harmondsworth

Freire P 1981 Education for critical consciousness. Continuum, New York

Friedan B 1963 The feminine mystique. Penguin, England

Frye M 1982 Willful virgin. The Crossing Press, Freedom, C.A.

Gee J P 1993 Postmodernism and literacies. In: Lankshear C, McLaren P (eds) Critical literacy politics, praxis, and the postmodern. State University of New York Press, Albany, New York

Gortner S R 1983 The history and philosophy of nursing science and research. Advances in Nursing Science 5(2):1-8

Goulding P 1993 Resuscitation. Royal Children's Hospital, Melbourne

Greenwood J 1984 Nursing research: a position paper. Journal of Advanced Nursing 9:77-82

Greer G 1970 The female eunuch. McGraw-Hill, New York

Gunew S (ed) 1990 A reader in feminist knowledge. Routledge, London

Habermas J 1971 Knowledge and human interests. Beacon Press, Boston

Hall J M, Stevens P E et al 1994 Marginalization: a guiding concept for valuing diversity in nursing knowledge development. Advances in Nursing Science 16(4):23-41

Harasym S 1988 Practical politics of the open end: an interview with Gayatri Spivak. Canadian Journal of Political and Social Theory 12(1-2):51-69

Haraway D 1988 Situated knowledges: the science question in feminism and the privilege of partial perspective. Feminist Studies 14:575-599

Harding S 1986 The science question in feminism. Cornell University Press, Ithaca, New York

Henderson V 1977 We've come a long way, but what of the direction? Nursing Research 26(3):

Hitchcock J, Wilson H 1992 Personal risking: lesbian self-disclosure of sexual orientation to professional health care providers. Nursing Research 41 May/June (3):178-83

Holly M L 1987 Keeping a personal-professional journal. Deakin University Press, Geelong

hooks B 1981 Ain't I a woman: black women and feminism. South End Press, Boston

Hull G L, Scott P B et al (eds) 1982 But some of us are brave: black women's studies. Feminist Press, Old Westbury, New York

Hunt M 1987 The process of translating research findings into nursing practice. Journal of Advanced Nursing 12:101-110

Johnston J 1973 Lesbian nation. Simon and Schuster, New York

Keefe M R 1993 An integrated approach to incorporating research findings into practice. MCN 18 March/April:65-70

Keefe M R, Kotzer A M 1988 Integrating clinical practice and research: a challenge for the pediatric nurse practitioner. Journal of Pediatric Health Care 2(6):275-280

Kemmis S 1985 Action research and the politics of reflection. In: D B et al (ed) Reflection: turning experience into learning. Kogan Page, New York

Kemmis S, McTaggart R M 1982 The action research planner. Deakin University Press, Geelong

Kennedy F 1993 Night duty rotation. Royal Children's Hospital, Melbourne

Kitson A L 1987 A comparative analysis of lay-caring and professional (nursing) caring relationships. International Journal of Nursing Studies 24(2):155-165

Lather P 1985 Empowering research methodologies. American Educational Research Association, Chicago

Lather P 1991a Getting smart. Routledge, New York

Lather P 1991b Post-critical pedagogies: a feminist reading. Education and Society 91-(2)

Lather P 1992 Critical frames in educational research: feminist and post-structural perspectives. Theory and Practice XXXI(2):87-99

Lather P 1993 Fertile obsession: validity after poststructuralism. The Sociological Quarterly 34(4): 673-693

Leineinger M M 1984 Care: the essence of nursing and health. Charles B. Slack, Thorofare, New Jersey

Leineinger M M 1988 Leineinger's theory of nursing: cultural care diversity and university. Nursing Science Quarterly 1:152-160

Lewin K 1946 Action research and minority problems. Journal of Social Issues 2(4):34-46

Lipman-Blumen J 1984 Gender roles and power. Prentice-Hall, New Jersey

Lorde A 1984 Sister outsider: essays and speeches. Crossing Press, Trumansburg, New York

Luke C, Gore J 1992 Feminisms and critical pedagogy. Routledge, New York

Lykes M B (ed) 1989 Dialogue with Guatemalan Indian women: critical perspectives on constructing collaborative research. Representations: social constructions of gender. Baywood, Amityville, New York

Maaresh J K 1986 Women's history, nursing history: parallel stories. In: Maaresh J K (ed) Nursing and feminism: implications for health care. Yale University Press, New Haven

Martin B 1992 Sexual practices and changing lesbian identities. In: Barrett M, Phillips A (eds) Destabilizing theory. Polity Press, Cambridge

Martin M 1990 Form-elation: an exploration of form in nursing. Myth, mystery and metaphor: the 4th National Nursing Education Conference, Melbourne

McCaugherty D (1991) The use of a teaching model to promote reflection and the experiental integration of theory and practice in first-year student nurses: an action research study. Journal of Advanced Nursing 16: 534-543

McClelland J, Ho S K et al 1993 The development of a clinical neonatal program. Royal Children's Hospital, Melbourne

McEwan J 1993 Nursing care plan project. Royal Children's Hospital, Melbourne

McLaren P 1988 Schooling the postmodern body: critical pedagogy and the politics of enfleshment. Journal of Education 170(3):53-83

McLaren P, Hammer R 1989 Critical pedagogy and the postmodern challenge: towards a critical postmodernist pedagogy of liberation. Educational Foundations (Fall):29-62

McTaggart R 1991a Action research: a short modern history. Deakin University Press, Geelong

McTaggart R 1991b Principles for participatory action research. Journal of the Participatory Action Research Network 1

Minh-Ha T T 1991 When the moon waxes red. Routledge, New York

Morarga C 1986 From a long line of vendidas: chicanas and feminism. In: de Lauretis T (ed) Feminist studies/critical studies. Indiana University Press, Bloomington

Morarga C, Anzldua G (eds) 1983 This bridge called my back: writings by radical women of color. Kitchen Table: Women of Color Press, New York

Morse J, Bottorff J et al 1991 Comparative analysis of conceptualizations and theories of caring. Image: Journal of Nursing Scholarship 23(2):119-126

Moyers B 1988 Myth and the modern world. In: Moyers J C w B (ed) The power of myth. Doubleday, USA

O'Reagan K 1992 A users guide to the Mental Health (Compulsory Assessment and Treatment) Act 1992. Department of Health, New Zealand

Oakley A 1986 Telling the truth about Jerusalem. Routledge & Kegan Paul, London

Oberg A 1990 Methods and meanings in action research: the action research journal. Theory Into Practice 29(3):214-221

Opie A 1992 There's nobody there: community care of confused older people. Oxford University Press, Auckland

Parsons C, Blackford J et al 1994 Multicultural Australia: nurses in action. Health & Community Services, Royal Children's Hospital and La Trobe University, Melbounrne

Parsons C, Street A et al 1994 Parental decisionmaking and therapeutic noncompliance: a study of cognition and action. Australian Research Council Small Project Grant

Pearson A 1985 Nurses as change agents and a strategy for change. Nursing Practice 2:80-84

Poland F 1990 Breaking the rules: assessing the assessment of a girl's project. In: Stanley L (ed) Feminist praxis. Routledge, London

Porter S 1993 Nursing research conventions: objectivity or obfuscation? Journal of Advanced Nursing 18:137-143

Raymond J 1986 A passion for friends: towards a philosophy of female affection. Beacon Press, Boston

Reason P (ed) 1988 Human inquiry in action. Sage, London

Rice P L 1993 My forty days. The Vietnamese antenatal/postnatal support project. Centre for the study of Mothers and Children's Health, Melbourne

Ridpath I 1985 Hamlyn encyclopedia of space. Hamlyn, London

Robinson A, O'Connell C 1994 Conflicts of practice confronting second line nurse managers in an A & E department. Accident and Emergency Nursing: an International Journal. In press (in two volumes)

Robinson A, Oxnam K et al 1993 A study into nursing children with disabilities in an acute care context. Royal Children's Hospital, Melbourne

Rose G 1993 Feminism and geography: the limits of geographical knowledge. University of Minnesota Press, Minneapolis

Rowland R 1988 Woman herself: a transdisciplinary perspective on women's identity. Oxford University Press, Oxford

Shea C A 1979 Action research: for nurses, with nurses. In: Clark C C, Shea C A (eds) Management in nursing: a vital link in the health care system. McGraw-Hill, New York

Smith G 1986 Resistance to change in geriatric care. International Journal of Nursing Studies 23(1):61-70

Smyth J 1986 The reflective practitioner in nurse education. Second National Nursing Education Seminar, Adelaide, South Australia

Spain D 1992 Gendered spaces. The University of North Carolina Press, Chapel Hill

Spivak G 1990 The post-colonial critic. Routledge, New York

Stanley L 1990 Feminist praxis. Routledge, London

Stanley L, Wise S 1993 Breaking out again: feminist ontology and epistemology. Routledge, London

Stein L 1967 The nurse-doctor game. Archives of General Psychiatry 16:699-703

Street A 1990a The practice of journalling: for teachers, nurses, adult educators and other professionals. Deakin University, Victoria

Street A 1990b Launching into the deep: dealing with doubts, dilemmas and despair. Embodiment empowerment emancipation: critical theory, reflectivity and nursing practice. Melbourne, February 15-16

Street A 1990c Nursing myths in action. Myth, mystery and metaphor. The 4th national nursing education conference, Melbourne, November

Street A 1990d Nursing practice. High, hard ground, messy swamps and the pathways in between. Deakin University Press, Geelong

Street A 1991 From image to action: reflection in nursing practice. Deakin University Press, Geelong

Street A 1992a Inside nursing: a critical ethnography. State University of New York Press, Albany, New York

Street A 1992b Cultural practices in nursing. Deakin University Press, Geelong

Street A 1992c Critical theory: making it work. Searches for meaning in nursing 2: cultural meanings and practices in nursing. Deakin University, Geelong

Street A 1993a The mad hatter's tea party: issues surrounding the practice of community mental health nurses using the New Zealand Mental Health (Compulsory Assessment and Treatment) Act 1992. In: Through the looking glass: the DAO conference. Porirua, October 19

Street A 1993b Here there be mermaids, here there be dragons. Mapping the terrain of feminist theory and nursing practice. Shaping Nursing Theory and Practice. La Trobe University, Melbourne

Street A, Walsh C 1994a Moving forward: the further development of nursing research at the Royal Children's Hospital. Royal Children's Hospital Nursing Research Management Group, Melbourne

Street A, Walsh C 1994b The legalisation of a therapeutic role: implications for the practice of community mental health nurses using the New Zealand Mental Health (Compulsory Assessment and Treatment) Act 1992. Australian & New Zealand Journal of Mental Health Nursing, June

Styles M M 1982 On nursing: toward a new endowment. C V Mosby, Missouri

Thompson J 1991 Exploring gender and culture with Khmer refugee women: reflections on participatory feminist research. Advances in Nursing Science 13(3):30-48

Tripp D H 1990 Socially critical action research. Theory Into Practice 29(3):158-166

van Manen M 1990 Beyond assumptions: shifting the limits of action research. Theory Into Practice 29(3):152-156

Wadsworth Y 1984 Do it yourself social research. Victorian Council of Social Services and Melbourne Family Care Organization, Melbourne

Wadsworth Y 1991 What is participatory action research? Action Research Issues Association, Melbourne

Walker K 1993 What it might mean to be a nurse: a discursive ethnography. La Trobe University, Australia

Watson J 1985 Nursing: human science and human care. A theory of nursing. National League for Nursing, New York

Watson J 1987 Nursing on the caring edge: metaphorical vignettes. Advances in Nursing Science 10(1):10-18

Webb C 1989 Action research: philosophy, methods and personal experiences. Journal of Advanced Nursing 14:403-410

Webb C 1990 Partners in research. Nursing Times 863(2):40-44

Webb C 1991 Action research. In: Cormack D F S (ed) The research process in nursing, 2nd edn. Blackwell, London

Weedon C 1987 Feminist practice and poststructuralist theory. Basil Blackwell, London

Wheeler C E, Chinn P L 1989 Peace and power. National League for Nursing, New York

Whyte W F (ed) 1991 Participatory action research. Sage Publications, California

Index

moral judgements, in nursing work 18
multi-skilling 23
multicultural families, nursing to, and
        the tyranny of niceness 36-9
multicultural myths 9-12
mythical nurse 3-5
mythical nursing team 21-2
mythical professional nurse 5-9
myths
    and culture 3
    and heterosexuality of nurses and
        patients 12-14
    and pre-eminence of medical
        research 14-16
    power of 2-3
    transcultural 9-12

negotiated decision making 158-60
New Zealand, community psychiatric
        nurses, role as DAOs 129-45
night duty roster problem 121-2
non-English speaking background
        children, digestive problems in
        112-13
non-English speaking background
        families
    communication difficulties 9-11,
        36-9
    PAR project 65-6
non-hierarchical participatory research
        xiv
nurse scholars, in participatory
        research projects 81
nurses
    and the tyranny of niceness 30-2
    approach to patient's bed 48-50
    as data collectors, in medical
        research projects 15-16
    continual interruptions to their work
        53
    work under public gaze 50-1
    work with parents in determining
        children's care 33-6
nursing
    and power relationships 43-5
    control myths in 16-18
nursing administration, myth over
        adaptability of nurses 22-3
nursing autonomy concept, distortion
        of 35-6
nursing concerns, as possible PAR
        topics xxiv, xxvi
nursing culture 1-3, 155
    and learning to cope with
        interruptions 53-5
    and trivial interruptions of patients
        and staff 55

changing through research 178-83
nursing educators, and the mythical
        professional nurse 5-9
nursing gaze 47, 48
nursing myths
    and feminism 7-9
    and nursing culture 3
    critical analysis of 6-7
    power of 2-3
    remythologising 18-25
nursing practice, use of journalling in
        147-71
nursing research
    as a means of changing nursing
        culture 178-83
    as non-elitist activity 182
    benefits of 177-8
    Centre for Studies in Paediatric
        Nursing xix-xx
    commitment to 175-7
    enthusiasm for 181-2
    reasons some nurses do not become
        involved 176-7, 180
    structure 88
    unwarranted feelings about 84-5
    what is it? 174
nursing research scholarships 90-1
nursing role
    and nursing culture 32
    in the caring unit 30
    representation of 45-6
nursing team, myths surrounding
        19-20, 21-2

occupation, and level of work under
        the public gaze 50
'open floor' occupations 50
orthopaedic unit, discharge education
        65
over-researching, of vulnerable clients
        100

pain, in young children, myth 18-19
PAR xi
    and problems of dealing in
        uncertainties 183-5
    and research method xvi
    baby example xi-xii
    background to the problem 125-6
    costs involved 79-80
    difficulties with rostering and shift
        work 85-7
    distinction from conventional
        research designs xxiii-xxiv
    findings 126-7
        implementation of 83-4
    funding and its implications 79-82